KT-501-538

Advance praise for *The Happy Birth Book*

'If you are having a baby, this is a MUST READ. Get the birth you want whatever path you choose. It IS possible to enjoy giving birth. This is all about empowering you as a mummy'

Davina McCall

'This is an amazing book. It will help you understand some complicated things about giving birth, but it is also so lively and understanding, with a lovely way of talking about feelings. Above all, *The Happy Birth Book* emphasises that you are the expert on you, reminds you that your mind and body are connected (surprisingly, this is often overlooked), and encourages you to aim high for a good experience. Full of information, realistic and not sentimental, *The Happy Birth Book* will help you work towards a good birth. It should be read by every woman having a baby, every partner becoming a parent and by whoever else is involved. It should also be read by anyone providing care around birth, including students'

Lesley Page, President of The Royal College of Midwives

'A practical, no-nonsense approach to ensuring you are fully prepared for the greatest adventure out there!'

Bear Grylls, adventurer and father of three

'I am thrilled that Beverley Turner and Pam Wild have put this wonderful book together. *The Happy Birth Book* will give you a straightforward point of view, help calm the worries you may have about giving birth and provide information that will enable you to make informed choices'

Tiggy Pettifer (née Legge-Bourke),
former companion to Princes William and Harry

C334087372

'Beverley Turner is at the forefront of a new generation leading birth into the future. Her passion for women's well-being, her common-sense and eye for humour emanate off every page. This book teaches century's old truths through a uniquely modern perspective. It will become a classic. It is a must-have for every pregnant woman and every midwife'

Professor Caroline Flint, midwife, NCT teacher and trustee, Past President of The Royal College of Midwives, and author

'This is a great book. I thoroughly enjoyed reading this no-nonsense guide to giving birth and what to expect. Beverley has the rare talent of being able to distil complex information into a format we can all understand. I laughed out loud many times. She's effortlessly combined factual medical information and good old-fashioned common sense. As a doctor who doesn't believe in over-medicalising the normal condition of pregnancy, I found her approach refreshing. Another important aspect of this book is that it reinforces the fact that the process of giving birth is a complex interaction between body and mind, and both have to be prepared. *The Happy Birth Book* gives great medical, psychological and social advice, which means you will be 110 per cent ready for the big day. I think every expectant parent – male and female – should be given a copy. And I have to admit that, despite being a doctor with a lot of experience of maternity wards, I learnt some stuff that blew my mind'

Dr David Bull, Medical Consultant, TV host and broadcaster

'This is such a wonderful book – reading it made us feel looked after and very cared for all over again. Having Pam as our midwife truly was the most wonderful and magical journey we have ever experienced. To feel understood is such a precious thing and the message that these two women share is such a strong and beautiful one for all of us – men and woman. Thank you, you really rock!'

Nora Kryst and Fran Healy, from Travis

'Becoming a dad can be really scary. This book will give you a head start. Pam Wild is an amazingly experienced midwife who gave my wife Carolin and I huge confidence to have two calm homebirths'

Matt Dawson, Rugby World Cup winner and TV presenter

'When I have a baby, Beverley Turner will be my Ambassador of Awesomeness'

**Emma Barnett, BBC Radio 5 Live
and BBC Woman's Hour presenter**

'Everything I needed to know, even some bits I didn't want to know. A brilliant guide for anyone wading through oodles of conflicting advice'

Helen Skelton, BBC TV presenter

The
Happy Birth
Book

Beverley Turner
with midwife Pam Wild

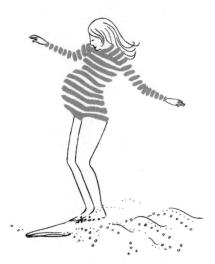

piatkus

PIATKUS

First published in Great Britain in 2017 by Piatkus

1 3 5 7 9 10 8 6 4 2

Copyright © Beverley Turner 2017

The moral right of the author has been asserted.

All rights reserved.
No part of this publication may be reproduced, stored in
a retrieval system, or transmitted in any form or by any means, without
the prior permission in writing of the publisher, nor be otherwise circulated
in any form of binding or cover other than that in which it is published
and without a similar condition including this condition
being imposed on the subsequent purchaser.

A CIP catalogue record for this book
is available from the British Library.

ISBN 978-0-349-41291-7

Illustrations on pages 275–8 by Emily Hamilton; all others by D.R. ink.

Typeset in Palatino by M Rules
Printed and bound by CPI Group (UK) Ltd, Croydon, CR0 4YY

Papers used by Piatkus are from well-managed forests
and other responsible sources.

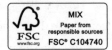

MIX
Paper from
responsible sources
FSC
www.fsc.org
FSC® C104740

Piatkus
An imprint of
Little, Brown Book Group
Carmelite House
50 Victoria Embankment
London EC4Y 0DZ

An Hachette UK Company
www.hachette.co.uk

www.improvementzone.co.uk

Disclaimer
The information in this book is not intended to replace the advice given
to you by your GP or other health professionals. All matters regarding
your health and that of your baby should be discussed with your GP.
The author and publisher disclaim any liability directly or indirectly
from the use of the material in this book by any person.

Beverley Turner founded The Happy Birth Club (formerly The Blooming Bunch) in 2013 to meet the needs of couples in West London wanting fun, informative and non-cringeworthy antenatal classes. She is perhaps best known for her work in the media as a journalist, TV presenter and host of her own phone-in current-affairs show on LBC Radio. Beverley sits on the Royal College of Midwives' Better Births Initiative team and chairs events for IMUK, Birthrights and Doula UK. She is also a trained psychotherapist and hypnotherapist, but she keeps this quiet in case people think she is a weirdo. She has three children and is married to Olympic gold medallist, James Cracknell.

Pam Wild was Beverley's own midwife and now works alongside her as The Happy Birth Club's dedicated midwife. Over 25 years she has delivered over four thousand babies in all settings: NHS hospitals, midwifery-led units, home births and the UK's first private birth centre. Pam is a passionate advocate of protecting women's rights and choices to birth where and how they wish – be that a water birth at home or a planned caesarean. She worked as an independent midwife for 17 years until 2017 while also providing NHS back-up near to her home in Wiltshire. She divides her time between there and London with her husband, Pete, and their four golden retrievers.

For every woman (and man)
who lets us be a tiny part of their
journey into parenthood.

Contents

Acknowledgements

Thank you to every midwife, doula, doctor and mummy who has inspired me to keep learning and listening so that I might help other women enjoy their pregnancies and births. I am immensely grateful, first and foremost, to Pam – without your tireless energy and encouragement, my love of this topic would never have begun. Rob and Kate at The City Barge – thanks for letting us traipse so many swollen ankles through your door and into your beautiful pub. Thanks to Marlene at The Little Gym – I love our collaboration; you do such great work. Emily Hamilton, illustrator extraordinaire – you are awesome, thank you.

Thanks to agent Sophie Lambert for your time and professionalism – knowing that you simply 'got it' made all the difference.

What would I have done without the team at Little Brown: Zoe Bohm, Jillian Stewart, Jan Cutler, Ella Bowman and Aimee Kitson? What a joy to work with strong, smart women. But not, of course, forgetting the men: Rowan and Andy at Soapbox PR – thanks for the laughs and for not running away when I talked about mucus plugs.

Huge thanks to all those who have generously provided their expert knowledge: Professor Donald Gibb, Shawn Walker, Victoria Cochrane, Gordana Petrovic, Olivia Southey, Jessica Scott, Hannah Cooksey, Lisa Opie, Chloe Dymond Tucker, Professor Greg Whyte, Rebecca Morley, Maggie Howell, Annie

Simpson and Vanessa Christie; plus the mums from The Happy Birth Club who gave their personal stories – your experiences will help others. Thank you.

I'm so blessed to have the finest extended family imaginable: Cal and Rick, Adi and Abi – thanks for being my very best friends and helping to create seven crazy cousins who adore each other. Thanks to my own mum, the indefatigable Nanna Joyce: you gave me the confidence to take ownership of my births, question everything and believe in myself as a mother. Dad too, the steady rock to cling to, who thinks his children are brilliant, no matter what we do, and is my favourite crossword partner. Jennie and John, you're the best in-laws anyone could ever ask for, and you made an excellent son. To Kat and Monika – you are Team Turner-Cracknell and without you the whole bloody thing would collapse.

Lastly to my kids: Croyde, Kiki and Trixie, your births were the best days of my life. Remember – who loves you? Mummy loves you . . .

And to James, my partner of 16 years: our life may be chaotic, busy and unpredictable, but thank God for you. Cheers for still being handsome, kind, thoughtful and (occasionally) really bloody funny.

Introduction
Why You Must Read This Book

Pregnancy, birth and the early weeks of being a parent are highly likely to blow your mind. It's the start of a life-changing journey that is best begun feeling joyful and empowered. I feel passionately that all mothers deserve a happy birth to set them onto the path of parenthood with a spring in their step and confidence in their heart. With the right preparation, such an event is entirely possible.

And yet it has never been harder to get the birth that you want; there has never been such fear surrounding labour or such high rates of unnecessary medical tinkering with female bodies. Reports of traumatic births are at an all-time high, postnatal depression continues to rise, and the UK has the lowest breast-feeding rate *in the whole world*. Women who endure a tough time emerge from hospital silenced by the phrase, 'You have a healthy baby, and that's what matters.' But, surely, a healthy baby should be the very *least* of your expectations in the modern world. If blokes gave birth, I can't help thinking that that would be their baseline request. (On top of that, they'd expect a midwife that they knew, a private bathroom and a 70in flat-screen TV.)

Of course, the mainstream media is awash with stories of 'births that go wrong' without ever mentioning the thousands of happy labours that occur every single day.

I believe that in birth – as in life – women should be encouraged to aim high. At which other times do we tell women to shoot for the low bar, just in case they're disappointed? Have you ever heard any of these phrases?

- 'Give A-levels a miss – you won't be able to cope if you don't get As.'
- 'You mustn't aim to improve your piano-playing – just imagine how distraught you will be when you mess up.'
- 'Yes, that bloke you met online might be gorgeous, but you must settle for Mr Average when it comes to marriage. That way you'll avoid any sadness if it goes wrong.'

All these notions are clearly nuts. Yet somehow, when it comes to birth, we tell women to aim low and to give up on any hope of an amazing day that they might actually enjoy. Decades of conditioning have told us to switch off our brains, pop on a medical gown with our arse showing, hop on the bed and hand ourselves over to someone with a name badge. You hear this submission to the inevitable in the language around giving birth: 'They won't *let me go* over 40 weeks of pregnancy', or 'I wanted a water birth but *they said I wasn't allowed to*', or 'I would have preferred a caesarean but *they said I couldn't have one.*'

The 'they' of which these women speak with such reverence are doctors and midwives – clever, educated, life-saving medics – but, nevertheless, they are not an expert on *you*, and all too often, they are operating in a one-size-fits-all system that simply cannot afford to view you as a single person with your own unique set of circumstances. Amazingly, too many of these medics do not even recognise the connection between the way you might *feel* emotionally and the way your body actually labours.

Hospitals are places of life-saving wonder, but their protocols can lead to a one-size-fits-all model that may not be in your best interests given your circumstances. Nobody will be deliberately attempting to sabotage your experience. But obstetrics has the largest litigation bill in the NHS, and it has tripled in the last decade to £1.2 billion during 2015/16 with 1,100 claims lodged. Because of this trend, hospitals commonly use a defensive-practice model of care – they will normally be over-cautious – which, in principle, sounds great. But in an effort to be hands-on, too many unnecessary interventions are causing needless complications which, guess what, can cause a poor outcome and, with a tragic irony, result in a huge legal bill. And so it continues.

This isn't meant to scare you. But forewarned is forearmed, and the good news is that such scenarios can commonly be avoided by knowing what questions to ask and which choices to make, in collaboration with – rather than at the bidding of – your medical team. If this sounds overwhelming, perhaps look at it as simply knowing that you have choices and can be involved in those choices.

Birthing women need time and compassion and their individual circumstances need careful consideration. If hospital staff do not have time to view you in this way and are busy wondering what a lawyer might say, a few questions or suggestions from you can make all the difference to having a happy birth.

In all honesty, even doctors and midwives themselves don't actually want you to rock up and hand yourself over to them and their sole decision-making powers. They don't want you to hand over the keys to your vagina and presume they're going to do all the driving. You can be active, involved and play the starring role in your experience of giving birth.

There has never been more conflicting advice at your fingertips about pregnancy, labour and parenting. This can leave your head spinning and your conscience troubled. Women have never felt more judged for their choices. Internet chat rooms inevitably become a refuge for worried mums-to-be. Sometimes, the advice found there will be supportive and factually correct – but, it's a lottery. I know many mums who have listened to the advice of a well-meaning stranger online to the detriment of their baby, themselves or their sanity.

The Happy Birth Book will lay out all your options in an easy-to-dip-into A–Z format. After all, you are intelligence-rich and time-poor. It will cut through the bullshit and give evidence-based facts clearly and openly, so that you can choose the path to parenthood that suits you.

Some books will dole out medical facts and then tell you to pop on the couch and do exactly what your doctor says. They fail to acknowledge that you are an individual and not a case study out of a medical textbook. Some of these books are also woefully out-dated. I only deal in evidence and facts – plus a dollop of experience and a particularly female type of common sense.

Some birth books are politically motivated: they want to change the system and expect you to take on that same campaign. Damn right, I want to change the system! I believe every woman should have a one-to-one midwife, whom she gets to know, on the NHS. But that's my fight to have outside of these pages. In this book, all I wish to do is to help you navigate the system that exists, know the questions to ask of your carers, and give you an understanding of the universal truths about birth. Because I believe you are strong enough to enjoy your birth wherever you choose to have it.

I feel passionately that every woman should get the birth that she wants: be that a planned caesarean, a home birth or simply using the birth pool in a busy hospital. I'm driven by a desire to see all women look forward to their labours with excitement, equipped to face difficult conversations but also trusting their medical professionals and able to draw on their own inner strength if twists and turns occur. I have no agenda other than helping you towards a special type of happiness that only arises from becoming a mum.

How to use this book

You can read *The Happy Birth Book* from cover to cover; look up certain words or, if your midwife mentioned a nuchal scan but you didn't quite catch what that means, flick to that section and digest it at your leisure. Some partners won't read a whole book about birth, so pop a Post-it on the bit about 'Partners' and put it by the loo. If your mum wants to help you with breastfeeding but can't remember how it was done in her day, show her that section. It takes a village to raise a child and it's so much more harmonious if you are all on the same page.

The Happy Birth Book will always be there for you – whether you're under pressure to make decisions about your upcoming labour or trying to manhandle massive bosoms with a screaming baby at 2am. This book will be an arm around your shoulder, helping you to breathe, encouraging you to smile and giving you the best advice available.

Knowledge is power. And, eventually, once you've had your baby, you too will feel the fearlessness that comes when you realise your body is just a-bloody-mazing, and you took control of your baby's birth – whatever that ultimately means for you.

Understanding the terminology of pregnancy and labour is absolutely critical to a happy birth, as it helps you to avoid feeling like a stranger in a strange land. Doctors have an obligation to make sure that you know exactly what they're going to do to you – and most of them do this brilliantly. But there are still some who will talk over you, using words that you don't understand. When these conversations potentially involve someone putting their hand up your precious lady parts, it's the sort of nightmare scenario that would have most of us waking up in a cold sweat. It doesn't have to be that way. Understanding when might be the best time to have an epidural, what happens during an induction or which natural pain relief options might suit you, can help enormously when it comes to working with your medical practitioners to bring about a great birth.

Of course, people will tell you, 'Yeah, right – your baby might have other plans', as though they are plotting to fuck up your big day. They aren't (they may, however, spend the next 18 years trying to do that). But I suspect that if things do take some twists and turns, you will be strong enough to cope – at least, you will be once you've read this book.

Consider this book a very safe pair of hands. I've worked in the birth world for over 12 years (it's like the real world, but people say 'vagina' *a lot*). I was inspired initially by having had a very happy first birth, when everyone around me was emerging scarred and distressed. I was also angry about this: I was no different from anyone else, so how come I'd had a birth in which I felt safe, in control and able to manage the (considerable) pain? But there was also tonnes of stuff I wish I had known: about how labour would feel and also about how life-changing being a mum would be. I wish I had known it was OK to say that, at times, being a new mum is lonely and boring and that it was normal to occasionally want to murder my husband. This book tells it as it is.

I also heard too many stories of women being cajoled into procedures they didn't want or treated without kindness. I guess it's primarily a feminist instinct – but if I could do something to help other women, then I had an obligation to do so. I learnt so much during that first birth – and even more so during my next two wonderful labours – that, like any great secret we discover, it is vital to pass it on. We shouldn't keep great news to ourselves: we should share it, be evangelical about it and spread that happy shit around the world!

I listened to many incredibly knowledgeable doctors, met

hundreds of wise midwives, read countless pieces of research and wrote numerous articles for international publications to demystify the notion of a happy birth. I've been fortunate to be asked to speak at conferences about my experience as one of the few media voices to speak positively about birth, and then, in 2012, I was able to establish my own antenatal education course in London, The Happy Birth Club (formerly The Blooming Bunch). By then, I had the greatest maternity minds at my fingertips and hand picked the ultimate dream team to pass on their knowledge, face to face, with couples expecting babies.

I slightly recoil at the description of me as an 'antenatal teacher', because it plays into the hands of the notion that pregnant women are like children needing to be told what to do. I believe every woman is an expert on herself and that her body *does* know how to give birth – you can't teach an innate physiological process. I merely facilitate conversations and encourage consideration of choices, explain definitions, relay possibilities, reveal likelihoods and encourage confidence, optimism and happiness.

By now, I've been privileged to accompany hundreds of couples on their journeys to parenthood. We discuss dozens of eye-watering topics, bust a huge number of myths – and laugh a lot. It's so easy to sum up what we do: we churn out happy couples who have happy births and enjoy happy friendships with the other couples that they meet. Simple.

This is by far the most badly paid and most rewarding work that I do. But I wouldn't have even started out on this path without one selfless, intelligent, compassionate woman.

Midwife Pam Wild sits alongside me at The Happy Birth Club. Thanks to her commitment to every couple, they coined the motto, 'Keep calm and call Pam.' I'm so lucky that three of the 4,000-plus babies she has caught in her 35-year career have been mine. She co-cared for me during my first birth alongside the legendary

Professor Caroline Flint. Pam then took sole care of my next two pregnancies. She is also now godmother to my youngest, Trixie, not least because that pregnancy was no easy ride – I discovered that I was pregnant with number three while my husband, James Cracknell, lay in a coma in an American hospital with a serious brain injury after being knocked off his bicycle from behind by a huge truck. Pam was the first person outside the family to know I was pregnant and she became a constant source of strength as I managed James's recovery.

Pam's client list reads like a who's who of famous vaginas (that word again – get used to it) but despite other mums that she has cared for, such as Davina McCall, publicly evangelising about Pam's skills, she has never sought publicity, never wanted her name in the spotlight and never asked for any praise. So, frankly, she's a bit cross with me for writing this book and putting her name on it. But we work well together and she has been through this book fact-checking, illuminating and correcting me when I got it wrong. Pam wholeheartedly agrees that there is a growing need for a no-nonsense, evidence-based, light-hearted handbook that couples can turn to for the most up-to-date advice.

As well as Pam, I am delighted to also bring you the insight and expertise of the team of experts that we use at The Happy Birth Club, including: obstetrician Professor Donald Gibb; nutritionist Jessica Scott; women's health physiotherapist Hannah Cooksey; osteopath Lisa Opie OBE; acupuncturist Gordana Petrovic; lactation consultant Chloe Dymond Tucker; and fitness expert Professor Greg Whyte. Plus, many other of the world's top experts who have generously written exclusive content for you.

So what are you waiting for – dive in, you're preparing for the best day of your life.

The Happy Birth Book will take you from this...

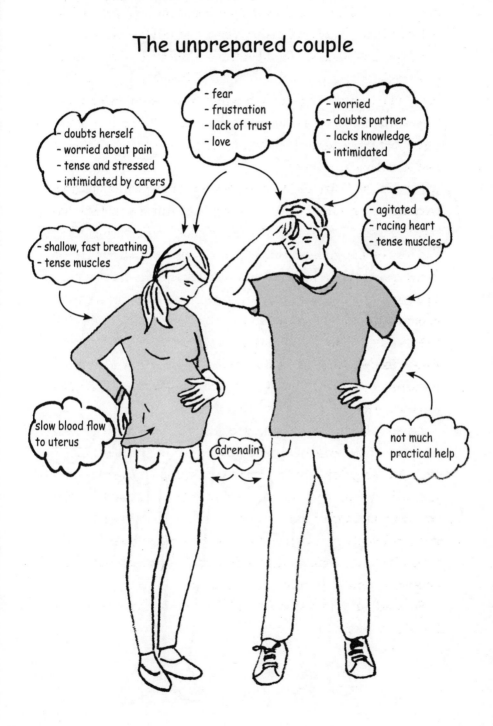

The unprepared couple

To this

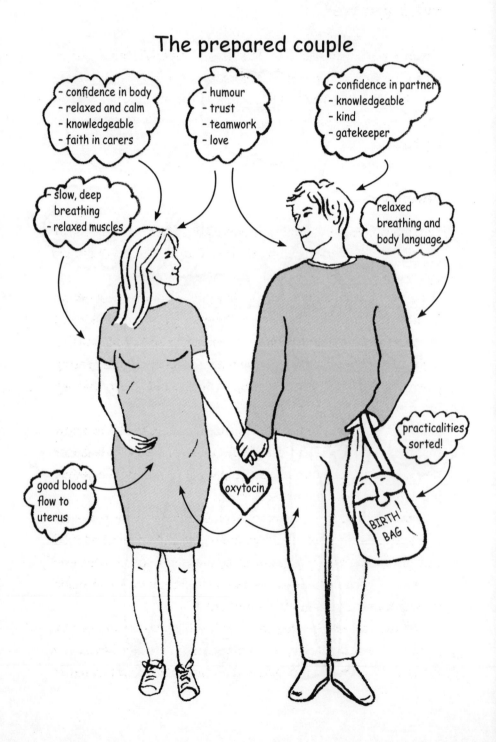

Who are we?

Given that we're going to talk about super-sensitive issues including your very precious lady-parts, you need to get to know me a bit. In the absence of being able to drink wine, I've put the kettle on, so let's sit down and I'll tell you a bit about me and my births.

Beverley

I am a birth junkie, shamelessly addicted to birth stories. If I spot you on the street with your bump or new baby, run. I will devour your stories vampirically, and you'll miss your train.

I wasn't always such a weirdo. Despite my mum's best efforts to make it sound OK, I grew up like most girls: fearing birth. I dimly recall a horrible secondary-school video of a woman with a huge amount of pubic hair giving birth on her back, and hearing playground chatter about 'tearing', which would burn into my mind at 3am.

The timing of my first pregnancy wasn't ideal, but I now know that there isn't a perfect time. If your own timing isn't ideal, fear not. Regardless of job or relationship issues, it will be the perfect baby. You will love them just as much.

Denial kicked in – I was too busy working as a TV presenter and journalist to think about what lay ahead. When asked if I'd thought about childcare, I burst into defensive tears: I'd cope fine without childcare thank-you-very-much! Pregnancy had made me sentimental (without the 'senti' bit).

But I was too chicken to give birth in a hospital surrounded by people I'd never met. I'm not saying that I'm a control freak (by the end of this book you'll know that's a total lie), but I wouldn't book a builder without three quotes and two recommendations. How could I risk handing the scariest day of my life to someone whose CV I hadn't seen? I didn't want to be making polite conversation with a stranger while I had the more important business of getting *that* out of *that*. It still floors me that the NHS expects us to share our most intimate moment with someone we have never met (but don't worry, I'm one of many women working on changing that).

Driven by fear and trepidation, I opted for the Birth Centre in Tooting, South London, run by Professor Caroline Flint, who turned out to be one of the original pioneers of active and water births. The location was a moderately sized 1960s' house with a couple of birth pools. Having St George's Hospital beside it felt vital to me as a first-timer. I didn't know if my body could do this.

The venue, however, wasn't as important as having a midwife that I knew. Caroline worked alongside Pam Wild, and I grew to trust them. For less than £3,000, paid in instalments over six months, we had unlimited access to both women, 24/7, for the duration of my pregnancy and until my baby was six weeks old. I was lucky to be able to afford this. My husband, James, and I decided that we would happily forgo other things for as long as necessary to feel safe and supported throughout this terrifying journey (see independent midwife, on page 212, for more on this).

With my first birth, I also took a Hypnobirthing course, which was regularly interrupted by James and I collapsing into giggles. But I learnt techniques to stay calm and breathe deeply. He learnt to be slightly more positive about labour. And we both learnt that we might not be grown up enough to have a baby.

Two days before my due date, I felt the warmth of breaking waters while at my laptop. It was the moment that a famous TV presenter was doing his first interview about a fake rape allegation (all that romantic stuff about spiritual births is lovely, but this is the sort of detail I remember about my labours). So I sat on the loo in our tiny flat from where I could watch the TV.

Eventually I called Pam. She said she would pop round later in the evening. And that was that. There I was in labour and the only person experiencing any drama was a TV presenter with an eye for the ladies, which I now know is exactly how it should be. Staying at home for as long as possible is vital in early labour.

Then, while wearing a giant maternity pad, I started to clean like an OCD sufferer on speed who has potential house-buyers coming round – classic 'nesting'.

The remainder of the evening passed in a warm, wintery daze as we lay under a blanket and watched a movie. I ate soup, went to bed and woke up about 1am with intense period pains that came and went in noticeable waves. Midwife Caroline Flint arrived and we had a cup of tea. She didn't examine me. Midwives who aren't constrained by dilation measurements on hospital white boards are free to use their other skills of observation, intuition and experience.

Soon, I knew that I wanted to go to the birth centre. James drove while I listened to the Hypnobirthing CD and Caroline followed. I was nervous – but felt safe: the most important state of mind for any labouring woman.

After some surprise vomiting, I got into the birth pool and uttered, 'Bliss . . . ' and it was. In retrospect it was also perhaps too soon, as I was still there six hours later. I floated on my back in the water, unable to use gravity to get the god-damn-just-fucking-pull-it-out-baby to descend. I was effectively pushing uphill. At one point I asked for gas and air, but Caroline said, 'You're doing beautifully' and that encouragement was all I needed to feel happier and for the intensity of the pain to dissipate. Weird.

Pam arrived and we decided I should get out of the pool. I'd been pushing for a couple of hours and needed to feel terra firma.

I was crying and saying that I'd changed my mind. I didn't want to be a mum after all. Could I please leave now? I couldn't do this. They wrapped me in a huge towel and I sat down on a birthing stool with James behind holding on to me. I have a photo of that moment. I've never looked more rough. But the relief of being in his arms is quite palpable.

In this position, the holy-crap-please-just-pull-him-out-now baby was emerging. Caroline was sitting cross-legged on the floor before me, kindly (*such* an under-statement) holding a warm flannel against my perineum. Sheer, undiluted terror at the playground tearing stories descended. This was it. I was about to be split asunder! Instead, the contractions simply stopped. The room was silent. My baby's head was partly out and for a split-second I truly believed that he would never exit and I'd spend the rest of my life walking through supermarket aisles as people pointed, 'That's the lady with the baby hanging out of her you-know-what.'

Pam broke the silence, 'Bev, tweak your nipple.'

What the fuck? This was no time for hidden-camera pranks. But I trusted her. As soon as my hand touched my boob, whooooosh! – a huge contraction, followed by a wriggly baby boy who promptly peed all over the great Professor Caroline Flint. In a move that would set the tone for my life as a mother, I apologised for his behaviour.

James cried. I cried. The baby peed some more. Pam told James to take his top off (benefits of skin-to-skin, apparently, not so that she could perv an Olympian's physique) and they checked me out. No tearing. Phew.

I couldn't process those last few moments in any way without feeling a bit shaky or upset, and yet utterly wowed that my body could do that; go through that and yet moments later, be sat on the sofa drinking the world's greatest cup of tea. It made me wonder why mothers aren't routinely celebrated as the goddesses we clearly are?

I was home four hours later and felt almost completely normal physically. It did, however, take me six years to do it all again. I really struggled with the identity change of becoming a mother: the guilt, the responsibility, the lack of freedom and lying awake asking, 'Why do I wear nothing but jeans and long-sleeved Gap T-shirts?'

Over the years, I had repeatedly reflected on this birth and wondered why it had gone so smoothly when my own antenatal classmates spoke in hushed tones as though they'd visited a war zone and couldn't speak of the horrors they had witnessed. Almost 50 per cent of this group had had caesareans that weren't of their own choosing. Thank God for caesarean births! But that seemed statistically too high to me. Our bodies were no different. So what – if anything – had made the difference? What could I learn for the next time? And what could *all* women do to get better, happier births?

By the time baby no. 2 arrived, I'd studied a two-year diploma in psychotherapy and hypnotherapy. The classes cemented my suspicion that our minds and bodies are inextricably connected. How we feel about ourselves, our setting and our companions is crucial.

A home birth was the obvious choice this time. Yes, I believed that my body would open-like-a-lotus-flower, etc., etc., but I also could not be even slightly arsed to go anywhere while I was in labour. Pam was back on board, and James accepted my argument that home birth was as safe as hospital birth. He was also rather pleased that if I did ultimately die on the living-room floor, he'd at least have his own fridge and Sky TV.

As a mother, I have to whisper this next bit, as our weird, patriarchal world does not want women to talk about good births, but the day of Kiki's birth was Totally. Fucking. Epic – the happiest day of my life. I would do it again tomorrow if I didn't have to raise the damn kid (kids, I'm kidding. Honestly. Mummy loves you – now run along, I might swear again).

The run up had been unsettling, as I was leaking water for a week, using up all my maternity pads and suffering from a bad case of trench vagina by the time contractions kicked in. If I'd been under standard NHS care that I hadn't questioned at this point, I would probably have been induced and started on a medicalised pathway. But, instead, I took control, asked questions and got a scan, which confirmed that the actual sack protecting the baby was intact. I had nothing to worry about. The leakage was from hind-waters around the baby's head. There was no risk of infection. I stopped worrying and carried on regardless.

Knowledge, ladies, is power.

I awoke a couple of days later with contractions. The rest of the morning was spent walking up and down the garden in slippers and a (regrettably) unattractive dressing gown. The hypnotherapy training worked wonders. I wasn't in Chiswick; I was on a beach watching waves in time with each contraction. I got a facial tan and Pam kept herself busy taking photos. I breathed Kiki out into the pool, off my tits on gas and air. She was out in time for lunch. It was Mothering Sunday and my parents arrived within an hour with six-year-old Croyde who brought flowers and chocolates. My dad kicked off his shoes to watch the football on TV and claimed it had been a decent day until Man Utd got beaten. My sister climbed into bed with me, we laughed at the pictures of Kiki making her way into the world and wondered if the passport office would accept a headshot of Kiki that included my excellent bikini wax. I had a daughter. She was beyond precious. She squared the circle. And I knew I'd simply have to do it all again.

An early miscarriage followed, but I was grateful to have two healthy kids. Then James was hit from behind by a 70mph fuel truck while on a bicycle and entered a coma with a near-fatal brain injury. He had been crossing America for a Discovery Channel documentary, and I flew to his bedside in intensive care in Phoenix, Arizona. At first they weren't sure if he'd wake up, then they were uncertain if he'd recognise me, and finally, categorical that he would never be quite the same again (they were wrong by the way). Ten days after the accident I discovered I was pregnant with our third child.

James was sent home an angry, unrecognisable version of the kind, funny father we knew and loved. His frontal lobes were smashed up – the bits that control personality, including the ability to empathise, which is a bummer for a sensitive pregnant wife. Pam became a constant source of support, reminding me that I was pregnant and had to also take care of myself.

This labour was odd because it stuttered and stalled. I just had to get through it before getting back to the difficult job of managing James and my other two children, who had been pretty hard work since the accident. I thought that I was relaxed, but I now know that being distracted by James's needs was choking off the hormone, oxytocin. In a constant state of alert, my adrenalin was on over-drive, and my uterus was on a white-knuckle ride.

There was almost no joy or excitement about this baby. I knew that even if he/she was born safely (my confidence in that was also shaken), James would still be his new, challenging self. In caring for him it already felt as if I had three children. I wasn't sure I could cope with a fourth.

I'd made no time to do hypnosis during this pregnancy, and Pam insisted that I lie down and listen to a Natal Hypnotherapy CD. I came to after half an hour of deep relaxation, listening to Natal Hypnotherapy's Birth Rehearsal CD, knowing exactly what to do. I wrote down ten pointers for James and showed them to him. He accepted my feedback bravely and promised to do his best. As he walked out, I felt my shoulders drop; my body felt lighter. Something had shifted. My mental block had dissolved. I picked up the phone to call Pam, my waters broke and we had a baby girl 90 minutes later, who James caught in the pool and lifted out of the water. It wasn't completely straightforward: there was meconium in my waters (meaning the baby had done a poo and might have been distressed) and she was also occiput posterior (rotated the 'wrong' way round) but she was born in the pool; it was pretty fast and definitely a happy birth.

I was done. No more babies. A switch had been flicked. My innate mammalian urge to procreate was no more. Pam helped me shower, held out my enormous knickers complete with massive pads to step into and made the tea. I shed a few tears in the shower that James was still not quite James, but I was soon tucked up in bed, introducing Trixie to her manic siblings.

All that I had suspected about the conditions required for a happy birth was confirmed that day: to feel safe, cared for and informed. Even if life is stressful outside the birth room, and even if things don't go exactly as planned, you can still retain faith in your birth attendant, remain confident that things will work out and have mental and physical skills to draw upon to continue feeling resilient – especially when you are part-way up a mountain and don't believe for one second that you can climb it.

Because, you know what? You can and you will. And a baby is a pretty great prize at the end of it.

A bit more about midwife Pam Wild

I wish I could tell you about all the famous vaginas that Pam has cared for, but she is annoyingly professional and discreet. Those who have publicly sung her praises include: actresses Jemma

Redgrave and Thandie Newton; Tiggy Pettifer (née Legge-Bourke), former companion to Princes William and Harry; Annabel Kindersley, formerly of the Dorling Kindersley, DK books empire; Fran Healy of the band Travis and his wife Nora; Ed O'Brien of Radiohead and his partner Susan; music composer and movie-score originator Joby Talbot and wife Liz; *Hitchhikers Guide to the Galaxy* and *Sing* Grammy-nominated director, Garth Jennings and partner Louise; Rugby World Cup Champion Matt Dawson and partner Carolin; TV presenter Kate Charman and actor husband Jason Durr. Davina McCall can be seen online talking humorously and movingly about the three home births she had with Pam.

But Pam would be the first to say that celebrity is not relevant. Every one of the 4,000-plus healthy babies she has caught was as important as the next. Some of the most moving stories she has told me over the years involve those women that she cared for who were living in poverty.

I could tell you that Pam continues to work in NHS A&E and maternity units, that she once assisted a triplet birth at King's College hospital, helped run a midwifery-led, 200-births-per-year NHS facility, 20 miles from the nearest hospital, where she would often care for up to six women at one time single-handedly but never considered it hard work. I can tell you she was the manager of the delivery suite at one of the UK's biggest hospitals, Guy's in London; and that she opted to become an independent midwife in 2005 in order to control her own diary and build better one-to-one relationships with couples.

But, really, all you need to know is what drives her. In her own words, Pam's job is to 'support women to do exactly what they want and make it happen'. She is a self-confessed oxytocin addict (I'll be explaining why this is so important later in the book).

She is busier than ever with The Happy Birth Club, but has one eye on the countryside and retirement.

How to get the most out of this book

The A–Z format that I have used should make this book accessible and easy for you to navigate. To make it even more straightforward to use, I've also made the pointers below for the most appropriate time to read each section on your journey towards birth and parenthood. These are merely suggestions – every pregnancy is different and the information that feels relevant to you can change on an almost daily basis.

Pregnancy These sections will be most valuable to you during the earlier stages of your pregnancy:

Acupuncture	Genetic testing
Alcohol	Home birth
Appointments	Hypnobirthing
Antenatal classes	Independent midwife
Assertiveness	Midwife (labour ward)
Birth plan	Non-invasive pre-natal test
Birth centre	Nuchal translucency scan
Diet	Obstetrician
Doula	Osteopathy (pain)
Epidural	Pain
Episiotomy	Questions
Exercise	Reiki

Getting closer As your due date approaches, you might find these sections most relevant:

Assisted delivery	Birth bag
Augmentation of labour	Braxton Hicks
Bed – get off it!	Breathing

Breech

Contractions

Cord clamping

Diamorphine/pethidine

Epidural

Fear

Gas and air

Gowngate

Heartburn

Induction – natural and
     medical

Internal examinations

K – vitamin

Labour

Microbiome

Movement

OP

Oxytocin

Partner

TENS machine

Positions

Water birth

After the birth Following the (very happy) birth of your baby, these sections will be the most useful:

Breastfeeding

Formula and bottle feeding

Guilt

Health visitor

Moro reflex

Returning home –
     the first two weeks

Relationship

Sex

Shut up!

Weeks two to four: looking
     after you and your baby

You – and your identity

Zzzz – sleep

Within each section, cross-references to other sections are referred to in bold.

A is for ...

ACUPUNCTURE

Although I used to be a bit sceptical about the benefits of this ancient Chinese practice during pregnancy, having seen many women try it with incredible results, and on Pam's insistence, I included an acupuncturist, Gordana Petrovic, in our antenatal care team.

Gordana has worked wonders for thousands of women, but she recognises that acupuncture is not a miracle treatment. It can be a powerful means of **natural induction** (see page 215) but is best used throughout pregnancy to get the full benefits. Some NHS hospitals now offer acupuncture as a means of getting labour started, so don't be afraid to ask if yours does. This is Gordana's expert insight into why acupuncture might be helpful to you, as well as some practical advice on finding the right practitioner:

Gordana Petrovic (MA BSc TCM) on acupuncture

Why use acupuncture during pregnancy? It works. Acupuncture is a part of the Chinese medicine model practised in the East for over 4,000 years. It is safe throughout pregnancy, provided you choose a qualified and properly trained acupuncturist with further training in reproductive and obstetric medicine to administer your treatment. Studies confirm its efficacy in pregnancy, especially in the preparation of labour and as an option for pain relief in labour. Acupuncture is used on site across hospitals in New Zealand, Europe and the UK.

How can I find a trusted acupuncturist?

Word of mouth is best, but, failing that, approach the professional bodies that have their directories of qualified and insured practitioners, such as the British Acupuncture Council, Federation of Holistic Therapists and British Acupuncture Federation, if you are in the UK. This will ensure you meet a qualified and insured practitioner, but it does not necessarily mean that you will get one who is experienced in pregnancy and pre- or postnatal care. Narrow your search by contacting practitioners directly and ask about their experience in this specific area of acupuncture. A good practitioner will give you some free time on the phone or in person, so that you can ask questions about their relevant experience and post-graduate qualifications. Valuable information can sometimes be given to you by your midwife, who may know of people or practices that have good results.

What should you expect in your first acupuncture session?

Acupuncture works best when an individualised approach to treatment is taken.

During your initial booking appointment you should expect a very thorough medical history to be taken: your pulse rates on both of your wrists should be assessed and you may be asked to show your tongue. This enables your constitution to be assessed according to Chinese medicine – this is the energetic state of your body and mind. The best plan for you should then be prescribed, and should take into account your age, previous medical history, general health, dietary requirements and lifestyle to maximise your chances of a smooth, pain-free pregnancy and a timely, natural delivery.

I would usually suggest weekly treatments during the first and third trimester, and more spread-out treatments during the second trimester; however, if this is not possible for whatever reason, adjustments are made to fit your schedule. Ask your practitioner if they are able to offer flexibility as part of their clinical work.

What can acupuncture help with?
First trimester During the first trimester, acupuncture helps the following:

- To reduce nausea and morning or all-day sickness. By being able to eat your meals without being nauseated, your energy levels will remain stable. Being able to eat healthily is a must when you are nurturing a new life.
- An ability to relax, if you continue to work and cannot avoid stressful people, work situations and events.
- To release endorphins, the feeling-good hormones, and lowers adrenaline, promoting relaxation. Your changing body's functions are regulated, allowing you to function without disturbance to your daily activities and family life.

Second trimester When you approach the second trimester, you might be faced with issues relating to the growing of your baby, and acupuncture is then invaluable to help with:

- Back and/or pelvic pain, either localised or distributed to other areas, such as in sciatica – it might start in the low back, and then refer to buttock and calf areas.
- Headaches, due to the changes in hormonal balance, might also be localised in certain areas, and then extend to your neck, shoulders and behind the eyes. As always and with any pain, it is very difficult to maintain daily life and responsibilities, and therefore restoring the homoeostatic balance to its best is very important if you want a healthy and symptom-free pregnancy.
- Sleep quality can often decline in this period, as your baby grows and you get more uncomfortable, especially towards the end of the second trimester. Having regular acupuncture treatments will help you to be free of pain and possible incidences of indigestion and constipation, which are often indicated during these times in your gestation. Indigestion very often prevents good sleep.

Third trimester In the last weeks of your pregnancy, your body goes through even more changes preparing you for the time when you will finally meet your little one; however, by now the symptoms of nausea and sickness most likely are completely gone and your hormones are more stable. Acupuncture helps to:

- Reduce stress, fear and anxiety related to the approaching birth date. This is very unlikely to happen if you had acupuncture during the first and/ or second trimester, because by this stage, most of your bodily functions, including stress regulation, are normalised.
- Reduce pain in the pelvic floor and low back due to the increased weight and the descending position of your baby.
- With the help of the associated technique of acupuncture, moxibustion, it can help turn your baby naturally without the need of medical intervention in cases of **breech** (see page 108).
- In the last couple of weeks, acupuncture helps to soften the **cervix** (see page 133) and to keep smooth, energetic oxygen and blood flow in the pelvis and the whole of the lower abdominal area.
- Once the baby is engaged, acupuncture can promote further movement down the birth canal and help to establish and/or regulate contractions – this is especially useful if your waters have broken but the contractions are at the start–stop rate and you are not progressing.
- Pain relief in labour with acupuncture is extremely effective, but this option might not be available to you if you are having a hospital birth, as some hospitals do not allow it, whereas others do, so it will depend on where your birthing is taking place. If you are having a water birth, acupuncture is used up to the second stage of labour.

Postnatally Acupuncture is used to speed up the recovery process, no matter what kind of birth you had, especially if during your vaginal delivery you had a tear or if you had a **caesarean section** (see page 115). It also promotes lactation should any issues arise with breastfeeding and by restoring hormonal balance. It can also reduce the incidence of post-natal depression.

Remember – acupuncture treatments will be beneficial to you whenever you take them up.

ALCOHOL

In the last 30 years, many of us (pregnant or not) have been drinking more units of booze, more often – fact. Since 2002 there has been a 91 per cent increase in hospital admissions for alcohol-related liver disease in women in England. Against this backdrop there has been a threefold increase in cases of foetal alcohol syndrome (FAS) since records began in 1998.

Almost 7,000 babies a year in Britain are now born showing signs of developmental damage due to their mothers drinking alcohol during pregnancy. According to drinkaware.co.uk, it is the leading known cause of intellectual disability. After decades of studying the condition, the medical world is now very good at identifying FAS's distinct facial features including: small and narrow eyes, a small head, a smooth area between the nose and the lips and a thin upper lip. But the effect of alcohol on embryos is not just cosmetic. It causes hearing problems, a weak immune system, epilepsy, liver damage, kidney and heart defects, cerebral palsy and low birth weight.

So why has this problem got so bad? Habit. Alcohol Concern reveals that adults in the highest income quintile are twice as likely to drink heavily as adults in the lowest income quintile – 22 per cent compared to 10 per cent. It is entirely normal for 'middle class' mums to offer a glass of rose at play dates (guilty, m'lord) or pour a G&T to take the edge off bath time. This softening of kids, booze and boundaries is a strikingly recent phenomenon born of relaxed licensing laws and a move towards a more European drinking culture.

Alcohol and pregnancy

Many women don't actually fancy alcohol in pregnancy – especially if nausea feels like a constant hangover anyway. You might carry around a huge amount of fear of harming your baby, and that causes you to be rightly cautious. But there is so much conflicting information about this topic that you may be confused about how much is too much.

It's probably second- and third-time mums who have to be mindful about reaching for a tipple at the end of a stressful day. You realise that your fears about your first baby's certain demise in your incapable hands didn't happen. It turns out that they are quite resilient. You reason that French women still eat pâté and Japanese women still eat sushi, and their babies do OK. Headlines repeatedly contradict each other, so you vow to ignore all this and listen to your body, but your instincts are now drowned out by a screaming toddler, a demanding job, a harried husband and ailing parents. So you sit down at the end of the day and tap the armrest like a smoker trying to quit. You miss the comforting ritual as much as the drink itself and decide that one won't hurt. And besides, the most recent news said that two (or was it three?) units once (or was it twice?) a week is OK.

It's just too easy to drink more alcohol in subsequent

pregnancies – one glass of fizz at a birthday party, became two (and the third as an 'oh, go on then' buck's fizz). Do we just lull ourselves into a false sense of security, having crossed the minefield of pregnancy and birth before?

Abstemiousness in pregnancy is Mother Nature's way of getting us ready for the enormous sacrifices that we will make thereafter. If we can't turn down a drink for the sake of a baby that can't make a choice, surely we need to have a word about our maturity as parents.

Although it is highly emotive, calls to ban pregnant women from smoking, drinking or using drugs tread on dangerous ground in terms of our own autonomy. All we can hope for is that better education leads to better personal choices, a stronger resolve and more individual responsibility. Drinks manufacturers still aren't doing enough to label food and drink for pregnant women, so without those reminders, do the right thing and look forward to the years ahead when you aren't pregnant in which you can enjoy a chilled glass of rose with a (relatively) clear conscience.

How much is too much?

The Department of Health recommends no drinking whatsoever in pregnancy. The NICE guidelines advise no alcohol in the first 12 weeks, followed by one to two units, once or twice a week without risk of major complications. But a standard 250ml glass of Chardonnay contains 3.2 units. A 125ml unit is a tiny glass of wine compared to the goblets we're used to pouring ourselves at home. If in doubt, leave it out completely.

Alcohol and breastfeeding

If you're breastfeeding, you will still have to wait a while to 'wet the baby's head' even after pregnancy. This is another area that is understandably under-researched. But there is some evidence that regularly drinking more than two units a day (250ml of wine or a double spirit) while breastfeeding might affect your baby's development. It is therefore recommended that you have no more than one or two units once or twice a week.

Your body metabolises alcohol at its usual rate, however, so think of the balance between drinking and feeding as similar to drink-driving. According to La Leche League, a 54kg (8½ stone) woman would metabolise a small glass of wine or beer in about two to three hours. This same-size woman might need 13 hours to eliminate a spirit such as vodka. So think about your size, what you are eating and also – crucially – timing.

Remember, also, that babies can be unpredictable. Even though it would probably do them no harm, do you want to find yourself feeding your baby 20 minutes after downing that Pinot Grigio?

If you have a big event coming up (such as a wedding at which you want to enjoy the free champers), then you could consider expressing your post-party milk and disposing of it down the sink, then use a previously pumped bottle in its place, or formula if you're mixed feeding. You may feel more reassured by purchasing some 'pump and dump' strips from an American brand called MilkScreen. These allow you to test your milk's alcohol content. (As far as I know, nobody is yet selling it as a healthy cocktail.)

Perhaps the best reason not to drink with a new baby is that you need your wits about you: there may be an unexpected drive to A&E or a last-minute dash in the car to get nappies. Plus, you may be emotional and tired; if you then throw a fractious baby and alcohol into the mix, there really will be tears before bedtime – yours!

AMNIOTIC FLUID

That big belly bump is not all baby – it's placenta and lots of lovely amniotic fluid: typically 800ml–1 litre of straw-coloured water by 36 weeks, which decreases gradually by the time you give birth. This is baby's personal, heated indoor pool, which they safely drink and then urinate in. (And who wouldn't want one of those?) It cushions your baby from bumps, and it aids the development of their lungs and digestion.

Hopefully, like most women, you won't ever really have to think about your amniotic fluid until it emerges, either when your waters break before or during **labour** (see page 232) or are broken manually during an **induction** (see page 215) or **augmentation** (see page 55).

When to be concerned

Too little amniotic fluid (oligohydramnios) or too much fluid (polyhydramnios or hydramnios) can indicate problems for you and your baby. Before your waters break there may be no symptoms of these conditions, and they will be discovered only by good antenatal care, which measures and assesses your bump. Scans are the very best way of knowing exactly how much water is present, so always ask about the water levels at each scan and examination.

Low amniotic fluid (oligohydramnios)

Sadly, low levels of amniotic fluid during your first trimester and in the early part of your second trimester can lead to an increased chance of having a miscarriage, or a stillborn baby. It can also cause growth problems and issues with lung development. If this is your experience, make sure you discuss all the implications with your medical team, remembering the BRAINS question framework (see page 279) to make sure you make the more informed decision about how to proceed.

Most cases of low amniotic fluid occur well into the third trimester, however, and although the situation still requires careful monitoring, the outcome might not be as serious. You may be prescribed bed rest and advised to drink plenty of water, receive an intravenous drip or be prescribed steroids if you are fewer than 34 weeks.

Low amniotic fluid can also cause labour complications. If your fluid levels are low, there's a higher chance of your baby becoming distressed and opening their bowels (passing meconium), into the remaining amniotic fluid. If the baby then inhales the meconium at birth, it might cause them to have breathing problems.

Low fluid might also cause the umbilical cord to be compressed by your baby during birth, which risks oxygen deprivation. Your baby will be carefully monitored, including continuous foetal monitoring, to make sure he's doing well, but a caesarean section might be necessary.

Excess amniotic fluid (polyhydramnios)

At the other end of the scale is an excess of fluid – called polyhydramnios. The cause is unknown but can indicate a genetic problem with the baby or its development such as a blockage in the gut (atresia) that prevents them absorbing the usual amount of amniotic fluid. A gut atresia would often require an operation after the baby's birth.

Polyhydramnios is more common in twin births or if the mum has diabetes (including gestational diabetes). If you notice your belly is getting large very quickly (acute polyhydramnios), contact your doctor or midwife. It's rare for it to happen suddenly, but it can indicate an abnormality with the foetus and increases your risk of giving birth prematurely.

For most women with polyhydramnios, the excess fluid builds up slowly. After 30 weeks this should be noticeable and picked up by your GP, midwife or obstetrician during an antenatal appointment. But trust your instinct – you will probably know if you feel there is suddenly too much weight from extra water.

It's worth remembering that the vast majority of women with polyhydramnios give birth to healthy babies. But request to see a foetal medicine expert, who will spend time assessing you through an ultrasound scan and will probably do a diabetes test also. Depending on the conclusions of this, you may wish to consider an amniocentesis.

How excess fluid might affect labour

- You might go into premature labour because of the additional pressure stretching the womb.

- Your baby may be in the wrong position, requiring a caesarean section.

- If your baby is in the wrong position, the umbilical cord may slip down into the birth canal when the membranes rupture, resulting in a cord prolapse.

- You might have an increased risk of bleeding after delivery.

ANTENATAL CLASSES

These were pioneered by the National Childbirth Trust 60 years ago and are designed to teach couples all they need to know about pregnancy, birth and being a new parent. They normally begin between 27 and 32 weeks, but that varies depending on your provider.

I resist the idea that women need to sit in a 'classroom' and be quiet while they are told how to birth their babies, but good, up-to-date, open-minded antenatal education that encourages questions and forges friendships must never to be undervalued.

Good courses get booked up well in advance, so make sure you don't miss out. Even if you don't want to pay a deposit upfront, register your interest and ask that they let you know if a course is almost fully booked.

Things to consider before choosing a course are:

- Do the people running the classes get back to you promptly?
- Is their manner welcoming?
- Do they cover everything from c-section to home birth?
- Do you feel you can pick up the phone and chat through any questions?

- Where does the group meet: a town hall, a pub or a practitioner's house? Where would you feel the most comfortable?
- Are partners invited to all sessions? Will you feel awkward if your partner can't make it to some?
- Who runs the group: a midwife, a trained mum or a host of different experts with various specialities?
- How big are the classes? Over seven couples might feel too many, but fewer classmates might reduce your chance to meet people you get along with.
- Are they held in the daytime, which means you'd have to take time off work? Although this is allowed by law, it may not help your relationship with your employer at a time when you might already feel awkward about your maternity-leave arrangements. Evening sessions might be easier for you and your partner to attend.

Your hospital might offer free, or heavily discounted, antenatal classes on the NHS. If they do, make use of them, but bear in mind that the couples you meet there may not live locally to you, especially if it's a large hospital. Having new-mummy friends within walking distance can be incredibly beneficial when meeting up for coffees once your baby arrives. If you have a caesarean you can't drive for six weeks and, even if you didn't, bundling a baby into a car and fighting for a parking space can be more tiring than a lovely walk with a pram.

Of course, with the advent of so many good websites, it's easy to assume that antenatal lessons can be taken online. But this misses the main, long-term benefit of pregnancy courses: to meet other like-minded women – or couples – going through the same emotions as you: excitement, fear, confusion and mind-bending wonderment. The support, advice and laughter you will provide to each other over the coming days, months and even years, is unquantifiable. New parenthood can be very lonely and isolating, so making new friends who will become your buggy buddies is a blooming good idea.

APPOINTMENTS

Perhaps it was the sore boobs, the late period or the foot-long baguette with extra olives that you wolfed at 10am, but however you discovered you were pregnant, your first thought was probably: *What the hell do I do now?* (followed by, 'is it too early for a piece of carrot cake?').

The chances are you went to your GP who – to your surprise – did very little except offer congratulations, pass on some leaflets about vitamins and book you in to your nearest hospital without much discussion about alternatives. These skilled professionals aren't doing anything wrong, but with seven minutes per appointment, they simply don't have the time to chat through your options and have no reason to know that there's a brand-new birth centre at the other hospital down the road that supports vaginal water births-after-caesarean using wireless electronic foetal monitoring.

Modernisation of maternity choices is swift, and so, through no fault of their own, your GP might not be up to speed. But fear not, this section will give you all the information you need.

All hospitals or local NHS Trusts offer slightly different schedules, but they will largely follow the timings set out below. All your appointments will be between 10 and 15 minutes in length, either in the hospital at which you are registered or at the GP surgery. If you opt for an NHS **home birth** (see page 197), you will still have all these appointments, but you might find that one of the home-birth team will see you at your home instead. You're also likely to see the same **midwife** or midwives (see page 243), as they tend to work in small groups. If you hire an **independent midwife** (see page 212) they will help you decide which of these NHS appointments you wish to have alongside their care.

Four to six weeks: finding a hospital

Once your home pregnancy-testing kit has confirmed that there is a bun in your oven, you can usually refer yourself online to the hospital in your area that you like the look of. This saves you a trip to the GP and you can do this when you are four to six weeks pregnant.

All you need to do is go to the informative, impartial, bang-up-to-date, evidence-based Which? Birth Choice site and follow the prompts to find the birthplace that you most like the look of (see Resources).

Then go to that location's website and follow the links to make your booking appointment. It really is that simple and avoids you sitting in a GP surgery breathing in everyone else's coughs.

As a courtesy, you can inform your GP's surgery over the phone that you are pregnant, as they will receive some correspondence from your chosen birth place.

Eight to ten weeks: booking appointment

Once you've referred yourself to a hospital or been referred by your GP, you will be receive a date for your booking appointment. This appointment happens at eight to ten weeks of pregnancy at the hospital of your choice. You won't necessarily have a scan at this appointment. But your height will be measured, you will be weighed, and you will have your blood pressure measured and urine tested, which might indicate complications such as pre-eclampsia or gestational diabetes. Three of four small bottles of blood will be taken for routine testing to establish your blood group, to check your iron levels, and test for syphilis, HIV, hepatitis B or any conditions for which you might be at higher risk, such as sickle cell disease. You will be given handheld notes and a plan of care (with options of additional support that might be needed in certain circumstances). You will also discuss any potential risks associated with your profession, such as exposure to chemicals or risk of harm that might arise; for example, a female police officer might wish to take an office-based position rather than attending incidents. You will be advised to discuss a revised risk assessment with your employer.

You will also be offered forthcoming screening tests for conditions including Down's syndrome via scans and discuss whether you would like to have any of them.

At this first appointment, the **midwife** (see page 243) (or occasionally an obstetrician, see page 249) will also talk through how the baby develops during pregnancy, what to consider in terms of diet and nutrition; **exercise** (see page 162) and **pelvic-floor** health (see page 269). They may tell you about **antenatal classes** (see page 35) in your area and maternity benefits, and they may even ask where you might want to have your baby: if you remain low risk, do you want to opt for the **birth centre, labour ward** or a **home birth** (see pages 68, 232 and 197)? Where would you feel safest? Remember that no matter how definitive your choices for where to give birth can appear, you are still able to change your mind closer to the date. Of course, if your pregnancy is more complicated – for example, if you are carrying twins or develop gestational diabetes – there may be a different unit that is more suitable for your needs.

Make sure you don't put your head in the sand.

Where you have your baby is absolutely crucial to having a happy birth (whatever that means to you as an individual) so why not refer yourself for booking-in appointments with several hospitals in your area? It is a little Machiavellian (and the hospitals don't need to know that you are actually doing this) but how else can you know which setting you prefer? Where did they treat you most considerately? Where did you get most time? Where would you feel safest giving birth? Once you have decided, make sure to call the location you didn't like and inform them of your decision. Easy.

Birth centres won't commonly accept you until later in the pregnancy once they know that you fulfil their low-risk criteria. Nevertheless, you can still pay them a visit, ask questions of them, register your interest and familiarise yourself with their location.

Eight to 14 weeks: nuchal, or dating, scan

This is commonly known as the 12-week or **nuchal scan** (see page 248) and is used to estimate your due date, check the physical development of your baby and screen for possible abnormalities.

It is a painless procedure where you lie on a couch, some cold jelly is squirted onto your belly and a plastic implement no bigger than a mobile phone is held against your belly to ping a moving picture onto a screen beside you.

The main purpose of this scan is to check that the baby is 'structurally' sound at this stage and to examine the nuchal translucency – or space in the tissue at the back of your baby's neck – as the size of this can indicate a genetic abnormality. If everything is within normal boundaries, you will go home with a snapshot of your growing person-to-be.

For the vast majority of women, this will be a happy day: seeing your baby wriggling around is an extraordinary moment, and for some comes the first news that there are two (or more!) babies-in-waiting.

Sadly, for some women, the news from this scan may be that there is no heartbeat, in which case your doctor will discuss your options and you may need support from loved ones or professionals to cope with your loss. The Miscarriage Association and Saying Goodbye are two British charities that do wonderful work in this area.

If there are problems with your baby identified at this scan, it can take four weeks for you to receive those results at your standard 16-week appointment. Consider a private scan if your budget allows. They are extremely thorough and offer results within the hour, which negates weeks of worry and means that if all is not well, action can be taken earlier in the pregnancy. At such an appointment (costing approximately £180) you will also have blood taken and spend up to half an hour being scanned with a foetal-medicine expert. These doctors have the luxury of time to talk through the details of your developing baby and will return your statistical probability of Down's syndrome within the hour.

Whether you are scanned on the NHS or privately, the statistical likelihood of your baby having Down's syndrome might lead you to request an amniocentesis, CVS (see **genetic testing**, page 188) or **NIPT** (see page 246).

16-week appointment

This might not be at the hospital but with your midwife at the health centre, so look out for a letter informing you of this. At this appointment, you will discover and discuss any anomalies (abnormalities) that were detected at your 12-week scan. Again, you'll have your blood pressure and urine tested, plus you will discuss your blood results. If you opted to be screened for HIV, syphilis and hepatitis B, these will be discussed with a specialist midwife (knowledge of carrying any of these viruses allows for medication that greatly reduces the risk of passing infection from mother to baby). You should get to listen to your baby's heartbeat with a foetal Doppler (a hand-held ultrasound device). You should be asked if you have any questions.

18–20 weeks: anomaly scan

This will take place at the hospital and is simply an ultrasound scan that checks the physical development of your baby and looks for anomalies. The main purpose is to check that there are no physical abnormalities. From 20 weeks, you will also be offered the whooping cough vaccine. The best time to have this vaccine is after your scan, and up to 32 weeks. But if for any reason you miss the vaccine, you can still have it up until 38 weeks.

If there are no immediately obvious anomalies, you will be sent home. You may then have an anxious wait to hear if the screenings throw up anything else unusual. But you will only hear from your doctor if there is a problem. This can be very stressful, so feel free to ring your GP within the first two weeks to check if any anomalies were identified. If it puts your mind at rest and reduces your anxiety, it's worth a phone call.

This is also the scan that can identify your baby's sex.

24–25 weeks

You will have this appointment only if this is your first baby. It might be with your GP or a midwife. They will use a tape measure to measure the size of your bump, measure your blood pressure and test your urine for protein. Listening in to baby should be standard.

28 weeks

Your GP or midwife will use a tape measure to measure the size of your bump, listen to the baby's heart with a foetal Doppler, measure your blood pressure, test your urine for protein and offer more screening tests; for example, glucose tolerance tests.

31 weeks

You will have this appointment only if this is your first baby. It will be with your GP or midwife. They will review, discuss and record the results of any screening tests from the last appointment, measure your bump with a tape measure, measure your blood pressure and test your urine for protein. A foetal Doppler can be used to listen in. They won't necessarily tell you the position of your baby, but this is absolutely crucial, as there are steps you can take if your baby is **OP** or **breech** (see pages 251 and 108). And if there's any significant doubt, ask for a second opinion.

34 weeks

Your midwife or doctor should give you information about preparing for labour and birth, including how to recognise active labour, ways of coping with pain in labour and your birth plan. Your midwife or doctor will review, discuss and record the results of any screening tests from the last appointment, measure your bump with a tape measure, measure your blood pressure and test your urine for protein. They can listen in with a Doppler so that you can hear the baby's heart. Again, ask for a full picture of your baby's position in the uterus. Is it head down or is it **breech** (see page 108)? If so, you still have time to try several methods to move baby around.

36 weeks

The midwife will measure your bump with a tape measure, measure your blood pressure and test your urine for protein. They should check the position and tell you if they believe it is **breech** or **OP** (back-to-back, see pages 108 and 251) as you will still have time to try to manoeuvre the baby into a more optimal position. If this isn't possible, you may not be able to use the **birth centre** (see page 68) and might be looking at a more medical model of care in the labour ward. You'll receive information about **breastfeeding** (see page 78), caring for a newborn, **vitamin K** (see page 230) and screening tests for your newborn baby. They'll also touch upon your own health after your baby is born, and postnatal depression (see **shut up!** on page 306). You should once again be able to listen to the baby's heartbeat. This is the session at which you can refer yourself to the **birth centre** if that is your preference.

38 weeks

The midwife will measure your bump with a tape measure, measure your blood pressure and test your urine for protein. Your midwife or doctor will discuss the options and choices if your pregnancy lasts for longer than 41 weeks. Astonishingly, many hospitals will automatically book you in for an appointment to discuss **induction** (see page 215) at 41 weeks. You can politely decline this offer at this stage.

40 weeks

You will have this appointment only if it's your first baby. The country's leading maternity hospitals conduct a scan before you sit down to discuss the results with your midwife. This is because the efficiency of the placenta, the amount of fluid around the baby and your general well-being should all be taken into account when considering if **induction** is medically necessary. Not all hospitals offer you a scan automatically, but you can ask.

Your midwife or doctor will use a tape measure to measure the size of your bump, measure your blood pressure and test your urine for protein. Baby's heartbeat will be listened to.

If your hospital doesn't automatically scan you (or even if they do) you will be booked in for an induction at 41-plus weeks. This can be made to appear as an inevitability. It is not. It's handy for the hospital to know who is booked in and who isn't. You can decline this assumed induction and tell your practitioner that you would like to see how you feel. Psychologically, you may feel demoralised by the assumption that you won't naturally labour, or it can add to the pressure you feel for the baby to arrive. Some women are desperate to get the baby out (particularly if they are suffering pelvic-girdle pain due to the rubbing together of the loosened pelvis bones) so, by all means, agree to the induction date, but be sure that it is what you want and not simply that which suits the hospital's protocol.

41 weeks

If you get to this stage, your midwife or doctor will use a tape measure to measure the size of your bump, measure your blood pressure and test your urine for protein. You will be offered a **membrane sweep** (see page 218) and be encouraged to discuss your options for induction if you haven't already agreed a date.

42 weeks

Despite all efforts to prevent this, and despite the keen and prolific use of tape measures, some women do find they are still pregnant at 42 weeks. You can still choose not to have a medical **induction**. In that event, you should be offered increased monitoring of the baby.

If you do decide to opt for an induction, you still have lots of choices about how this will work.

What else do I need to know?

These medical appointments are important and will go some way to checking that you and your baby are physically healthy. But there is so much more you can do to increase your general health and happiness during pregnancy: good **antenatal classes** (see page 35), **Hypnobirthing** (see page 206), **exercise** (see page 162), hiring a **doula** (see page 150) or **independent midwife** (see page 243).

◼ ASSERTIVENESS

Being able to articulate how you are feeling and expecting others to communicate effectively with you in labour can make all the difference between a good and bad birth. Research by the charity Birthrights confirmed that women who feel negatively about their births do not complain about 'pain' but they talk about 'not being listened to', feeling 'dehumanised' and 'helpless'. Second-time mums who join my course, often cry and use the language of disempowerment: 'I didn't know what they were doing', 'Why didn't they give me their names before they touched me?'

This stuff makes me cross, but fear not, there is a lot you can do – and it starts by being assertive. This is not easy when you might feel uncertain about a health-care system you are unfamiliar with, scared of birth or even just worried about your job. But, at some point, you will need to clearly and calmly make yourself understood by someone playing a vital role in the life of you and your baby.

What does being assertive mean?

Being assertive is simply a way of talking (and using body language) in which you maintain respect, satisfy your needs and defend your rights without manipulating, dominating or controlling others. It is a skill that is rarely taught, but it is always valuable, particularly during pregnancy when deciding your options, at the birth itself or afterwards, when receiving care from midwives or health visitors.

It is particularly important at times when we must 'defend our space' – sometimes literally (especially in pregnancy) but also in a more abstract way, especially when you are a new mother; for example, you might not wish to receive a vaginal examination (this can be vital if, for example, you are a sexual-abuse survivor) or perhaps you need the words to placate a well-meaning mother-in-law who is suggesting that you let your baby sleep in the wrong position. All such scenarios are likely to go more smoothly with fewer people becoming upset if you can be assertive rather than angry or submissive.

Yet, in everyday life, it can be really tricky to communicate without falling into these two traps. When you're angry, fearful or frustrated, it is especially hard to find the right words accurately, kindly and succinctly. So we freak out and yell at our partners before slamming a door, or we retreat into our shells, silenced and submissive. It is difficult to speak accurately while under stress, but it is not impossible, and a few tips can really help.

A common scenario

Kate is having a meeting with a midwife who wants to book an induction before her due date. Kate would prefer to wait and see what happens rather than feel she is under time pressure. Psychologically, this feels important to her. But she is meeting resistance by the midwife on duty that day.

Aggressive stance Kate's arms and legs are crossed with her body angled away. Her shoulders are high. She is talking loudly, but even smiles a bit as a way to disguise her anger, which undermines the message she wishes to convey.

KATE: You don't seem to be listening. You have a system, and I get that, but I'm not going to have you force me into it.

The midwife is likely to feel attacked and may become defensive or further entrenched in her determination that this woman obeys the system.

Submissive stance Kate's shoulders are slumped, her hands are upturned in surrender and her head is to one side. She sighs and looks to the floor. Her voice is quiet and sing-song.

KATE: OK then, if I must. It's probably for the best.

The midwife can fulfil her department's requirements but is unaware that the mother-to-be is unhappy (most midwives want to know if you are unhappy so that they can help). Kate feels helpless and tearful. She didn't want this to happen, but now she feels that she doesn't have any choice.

Assertive response Kate sits with both feet on the floor, facing the midwife squarely, sitting up straight but with a slightly forward lean. She has an 'open' position with neither arms nor legs crossed and looks directly into the midwife's eyes but with occasional glances away, which communicates an intensity of purpose without trying to overpower her with aggression. The body language suggests respect towards the midwife.

KATE: I can see that there is a system in place that must be
        necessary in such a big hospital. But I'd feel much happier
        if we could wait until my due date before discussing
        inductions. For me, that would feel like pressure and I'm
        keen to avoid that.

Then she is silent. The silence is necessary to allow the midwife to consider what she has just heard. It would be tempting to witter on here for most of us, to fill the awkward silence. But this is important to Kate and she could undermine her case if she didn't let the midwife respond. The chances are that she will be met with agreement. Or, as is often the case after assertive statements, she may be met with a defensive reaction, such as,

MIDWIFE: Well . . . I've got a job to do, I'm afraid, and this is the
          way it works here. So shall we say the 28th?

It would be so easy now to get angry! But Kate takes a deep breath, nods and tries to 'reflect back' to the midwife what she has heard:

KATE: You feel that there is no way around the system? [Waits.]

MIDWIFE: Obviously. Well, it's your choice but the risks to your baby increase if you go overdue. [Her pen is poised over the diary to schedule the induction.]

KATE (who has researched all the risks and knows this to be an exaggeration): You're worried that my baby might come to harm if we don't schedule the induction today?

MIDWIFE: Yes. [laughing to lighten the mood] If every woman came in here demanding that we don't schedule inductions we'd be in all sorts of trouble! Now, let's just put it down for the 28th and see what happens shall we?' [Writing in book.]

KATE: I prefer not to agree to that. I appreciate your concerns for me and my baby, but I am choosing not to commit to a date at this stage. I'm sure you respect my freedom to make that choice.

In an ideal world, these kinds of conversations would never happen. But they do. And it's a good idea to be prepared for them.

Tips for remaining assertive

- Breathe deeply before speaking.
- Be equipped with written-down facts or questions.
- Vent any anger at a trusted companion before the meeting so that it is out of your system.
- Try to avoid 'You' sentences, which can make people feel defensive, and use 'I' instead.
- Don't get sidetracked into small talk. Keep your goal in mind.
- Listen for phrases such as 'we should' and 'our choice' when having difficult discussions with medics. Ultimately, it is *your* body and *your* decision.

- Take ownership; don't say, 'They won't let me', but use 'I've decided to' instead; it makes a difference to how you feel.
- Never be afraid to voice your opinion: it's your body, your birth, your baby. You should be at the centre of all decisions.

Throughout your pregnancy it's crucial to remember that *you* and your birth are important. Your experience is important. A healthy baby is not 'all that matters' (see **shut up!** page 306). Your birth stays with you forever and can make a big difference to how you feel about being a mum and – possibly – how you feel towards your baby.

Jenna's story

I had imagined giving birth in the birth centre and my contractions started gently, but I was turned away for being 'only' 3cm dilated. When I returned I was 7cm and all was going to plan. But after pushing in the pool for three hours, the staff decided that I needed to go to the labour ward. The decision had been made for me. I felt helpless. But never mind, our baby needed to be safe, and so did I. I pushed negative feelings aside and was scooted in a wheelchair at midnight to the labour ward and into an assessment room – which had at least ten new professional faces in it. There was a lot of preparation and various types of medical equipment. Suddenly, the double doors were flung open and in marched a short lady with bobbed hair. She had an air of superiority about her, and she marched straight towards my vagina, spread open my legs and began delving around! No introduction, and no acknowledgment of the surrounding staff, all of whom appeared to be in awe of her. I was verging on rage. 'That's it! Everyone STOP!' I yelled. 'Tell me who you are, and what you want me to do, and I'll do it. But please, talk to me. Tell me what you need, give me a second to think and prepare myself. I can help, just work with me.'

My tone was strong, angry in fact, but I felt passionately that I needed to be involved in the process, to be included – not ignored – however potentially serious the circumstances. I was conscious, they needed to talk to me. I was not about to get excluded emotionally or otherwise from my own experience of giving birth.

I was spoken to. The room then felt comparatively relaxed and we all worked together to have an assisted delivery with epidural, forceps and episiotomy, in a way that involved me completely. Staff talked to me, explained their plans and reasoning, and I felt emotionally far more secure. In that moment I had seized back events that seemed to be spiralling out of my control.

Many of the staff were excellent that day, but this is an example of what can happen in busy wards. Tell medical staff what you need (they are not mind readers), encourage empathetic and effective communication, and participate fully in your birth experience and the decisions involved.

We named our daughter Boadicea. We want her to be strong, to have a voice, and to be resilient and empowered in life. Start with a strong name and hopefully, with support, the rest will follow.

ASSISTED DELIVERY

This might sound like you're collecting your baby from the Post Office, but it basically means that an obstetrician (or occasionally a **midwife**, see page 243, for straightforward ventouse delivery), will work closely with you so that you can meet your baby sooner rather than later. You're likely to be offered an assisted delivery if your labour has been long, you're exhausted and there is reason to believe your baby would benefit from being out in the world; for example, if their heart rate indicates distress.

Depending on the position of baby and therefore how much and which parts of the head can be reached, the obstetrician will suggest either a kiwi cap (formerly called a 'ventouse') or forceps (see below). The kiwi cap is normally the first choice, as it carries fewer risks to you and your baby. It fits via suction onto the visible part of the baby's head and the doctor pulls the attached string as you push. The fontanelle bones in a baby's skull are soft and malleable, so don't worry if the cap gives your baby a rather odd-looking cone-head for a few hours or days – I promise she won't look like that when she walks down the aisle.

Even at this point, you still have choices, and your consent will still need to be sought for any procedures, so make sure you know exactly what you are agreeing to; for example, do not be afraid to insist that the most experienced doctor on the ward conducts a forceps procedure. Forceps are perfectly safe in the right hands under correctly assessed conditions. Problems arise when incompetence meets metal. It is hard to be assertive in those situations – but don't be fobbed off. The midwife in charge and the midwife caring for you should also be in the room and can help you navigate that discussion.

Forceps

Forceps are like rather silver salad servers. They fit around the baby's head and are more likely to be accompanied by a side-order of **episiotomy** (see page 161). At least one in 20 babies is delivered using forceps. I think that this figure is far too high, because it indicates that too many women are not being cared for to avoid this outcome, such as being upright, relaxed and not in need of an epidural. Rates of forceps use vary enormously between hospitals. You can ask how often they are used when deciding on your place of birth. They are almost non-existent now in America due to the litigation risks that they carry.

In the UK, however, there are still many times when forceps are deemed necessary due to a baby's position. It is best practice to be in surgery for a forceps delivery with good epidural pain relief on board so that if it is unsuccessful, a c-section can be swiftly carried out. You will have your feet in stirrups but should be sitting at a slightly upright angle to aid pushing; however, a confident and experienced obstetrician who believes that a forceps delivery will be swift and successful might decide to remain on the labour ward. You might find that you prefer this, as it can be less frightening than being wheeled into theatre. You can express in your **birth plan** (see page 71) that you do not want forceps to be used and that, in the event of such a choice, you would prefer a c-section.

Your feelings after an assisted delivery

Research by the charity Birthrights shows that the largest percentage of women who feel unhappy about their birth are those who had an assisted delivery (not, as may be expected, an emergency c-section). Some find it traumatic, which can mean having to start motherhood with a troubled mindset. Women can feel that they failed or had those last few moments taken away from them in a brutal manner. These women can then be told, 'You have a healthy baby and that's all that matters.' It doesn't help that the notes accompanying an assisted delivery will often record this as 'poor maternal effort'. If you see this on your notes, you are allowed to despair (or laugh out loud!) at this use of ancient, misogynistic terminology. Then try not to give it a second thought. In the coming years, when you've fed your child Coco Pops for dinner (again) and cleaned their school blouse with a wet wipe, you'll realise a full understanding of the phrase, 'lack of maternal effort'.

Don't accept being told to **shut up!** (see page 306) if you find it tough to shake off the negative feelings. Talk it through and consider looking through your notes with a midwife.

AUGMENTATION OF LABOUR

Augmentation of labour is the process of using drugs to stimulate the uterus, thereby increasing the frequency, duration and intensity of contractions. Unlike an **induction** (see induction – medical, page 220), it is only used once your waters have broken or labour has started but stalled.

The World Health Organization recognises that prolonged labour is 'an important cause of maternal and perinatal mortality and morbidity'. In other words, once labour has spontaneously started, it's in everyone's best interests to make sure that it continues.

Once your waters have broken, you're at risk of developing an infection in the uterus and so you will have between 24 and 72 hours to labour depending on your hospital's protocol.

Syntocinon is the standard augmentation drug of choice; it is an artificial version of **oxytocin** (see page 257) and is administered via a drip.

If your cervix is already 'favourable' Syntocinon does the required job of speeding labour along. But if your cervix is tightly closed, administering Syntocinon is a bit like squeezing an unopened plastic lemonade bottle for several hours without loosening the lid. You will become tired, your baby may become distressed, but birth won't be imminent.

For this reason, those hospitals that are ahead of the curve, will offer a drug called prostaglandin gel (even if your waters have broken) to help you along. This is inserted into the vagina to soften the cervix and can work well alongside a subsequent infusion of Syntocinon. But not every hospital will automatically offer this, so ask. As with all drugs, too much Syntocinon carries risks to the mother, so doctors can only use it relatively sparingly.

If your labour is augmented, the stronger than normal contractions caused by the Syntocinon can put pressure on the baby – especially if the cord becomes compressed – which may cause him to pass meconium (do a poo) or compromise his heart rate.

A slow labour is hard to define in terms of hours – it largely relates to how you and your baby are coping; the frequency/regularity of contractions and the speed of dilatation. Only you and your medical team can decide if your labour is progressing too slowly given your individual circumstances.

The reasons a labour might be prolonged

Common causes of a prolonged labour include inefficient uterine contractions, an abnormal position of the baby, or problems with the mum's soft tissue/pelvis (such as **epidurals** – page 155 – which soften the pelvis tissue preventing the usual resistance against the baby's head to allow its rotation). But identifying the exact cause of a slowly progressing labour can be challenging and is much harder for midwives who are supporting a woman whom they haven't cared for throughout the pregnancy.

If your labour is stalling, you might hear the clinical assessment that you are 'failing to progress'. This term is so negative and demoralising for women that there is little else I can advise other than to laugh in the face of this arcane Victorian language, a hangover from patrician medics writing textbooks. I can honestly say that I have never met a woman who 'failed' to give birth – but I have met many who have been 'failed' by the conditions in which they are expected to give birth. It's a bloody massive difference.

However, 'failure to progress' (ha! See, I'm laughing) has become one of the leading indications for a **caesarean** section (see page 115), particularly for first-time mothers. Of course, amidst growing concern that c-sections are performed too soon too often, The World Health Organization does encourage doctors to explore less invasive interventions that increase the chances of a vaginal birth.

Natural or medical?

A greater understanding of the role of **oxytocin** and the importance of a homely birth environment (such as those created in **birth centres**, see page 71, and at **home births**, see page 197) means that more health workers will now consider natural methods to encourage labour, rather than reaching for a drip or a water-breaking hook.

It is very difficult to offer any specific advice about when medical augmentation is a good idea. Every individual case is different, and the decisions must always be taken as part of a much bigger picture. Your doctor is highly likely to be making the right decision for you, but challenge him or her to explain their course of action. Consider using the BRAINS acronym (see page 279). You may meet 'we' language assuming consent, such as 'This is what we want to do', or 'We're going to move things along now', but remember, you always have a choice and must agree to any procedures.

If there is any concern about the well-being of your baby in a prolonged labour but you still want to aim for a vaginal birth, it should be possible to take a tiny foetal blood sample from your baby's head to check her pH value and thereby detect if she remains well oxygenated. This can be tricky if you're only 2–3cm dilated, but if you're 8 or 9cm, then it should be straightforward. This information can then be factored in: do you continue with the Syntocinon or opt for a **caesarean** birth?

What can you do to help labour get moving?

- Go for a walk. Getting upright, out in the fresh air and in a less pressurised environment might be just what you need.
- Acupuncture – some hospitals have this available on maternity wards.
- Acupressure – you can self-administer this.
- Lie down in a quiet room and listen to a Hypnobirthing download. Breathe deeply and try to identify any anxieties that are weighing on your mind, then put them in a virtual hot-air balloon and watch them float away.
- Get your **oxytocin** flowing by requesting some privacy

and having a cuddle with your partner. Clitoral and nipple stimulation gets oxytocin flowing. Full marks if you can even manage an orgasm! (No marks are attributable to your partner. This is not their moment.) (If your birth partner is your mum, best mate or doula, I suggest you skip this bit.)

- Bounce on a birth ball.
- Sniff clary sage aromatherapy oil.

If labour still isn't motoring, what then?

Position of baby Is the midwife 100 per cent certain that it isn't **breech** (see page 108) or **occiput posterior** (in a back-to-back position – see page 251)? Ask for a mobile mini-scanner to be brought to the bed if there is any doubt whatsoever about the position and presentation.

Size Is your baby known to be particularly big? Might that be a factor?

Time How long have you already laboured for and how long do you feel you can go on for? If an internal examination establishes that your cervix is still not favourable (it is closed, hard and long) and you have already been labouring for 12 hours, can you face another 12 hours on a drip that might ripen your cervix but won't necessarily dilate it, despite the intense contractions you will feel? By that point, you may become exhausted and your baby could also become distressed by artificially strong uterine contractions. Is it best to opt for a c-section?

Previous labours Is this your first or second baby? If it's your second, the chances are that a small amount of the drug

Syntocinon, which is administered through a drip, will 'remind' your uterus what to do. If it's your first, it may not have the desired effect.

These more complex twists on your birth journey can prove crucial, and it's at times like this that having an advocate alongside (such as a doula or a midwife with whom you've built a relationship) can be a godsend.

The WHO states 'while interventions within the context of augmentation may be beneficial, their inappropriate use can cause harm. Besides, unnecessary clinical intervention in the natural birth process undermines women's autonomy and dignity as recipients of care and may negatively impact their childbirth experience.' Remember, there is no medical body on the planet that knows its stuff like the WHO. When it speaks, we should listen.

Of course, one of the most important things a labouring woman needs is time: time to relax, time to breathe, time to see what her body will do if left alone. Sadly, in some busy settings, this isn't always possible, and medics do want to reduce your risk of getting an infection if your waters have gone.

Timing is everything when it comes to helping labour along: intervene too early and it might be unnecessarily painful and still prevent you from giving birth vaginally; too late and your uterus (and you) might already be too exhausted to cope.

Your medical support will help you make an informed choice about the direction of your labour. Ask them to explain and justify their plans. But remember that you can state that you'd prefer to opt for an abdominal birth/**caesarean section** (see page 115) rather than a prolonged augmentation at any stage.

Darielle's story

My waters broke at 35 weeks on my last day in the office. I was bundled into a taxi and while on the way to hospital I spoke to midwife Pam who I'd met at The Happy Birth Club. She knew that my mum laboured quickly and we had to factor that in. She explained what might happen next and gave me some tips on how to communicate with the hospital. After being examined, the doctor said that he thought augmentation was the safest way to proceed. But my waters had literally just broken. I wanted to give my body an opportunity to do what it was supposed to do – I just needed a bit of a time.

The doctor wasn't entirely happy with my decision, but I was checked over. I was fine, baby was fine, so, firm in my stance, I was 'given' 12 hours. I wanted to find a park (not easy in central London) to make the walk a bit more pleasant. But all my husband and I found was a huge cemetery in which we spent hours walking up and down (looking at possible baby names on the gravestones). I could feel dull period pain-like aches coming and going.

It was dark now and we walked to the gates, only to find them locked! There was no way I could climb over them! Luckily, my husband found a warden's number and when he told him I was about to give birth in his graveyard he got there pretty quickly.

Arriving back at the hospital, I was told that nothing would happen soon; my husband was sent home and I was instructed to keep on walking. I spent a couple of spooky hours wandering the deserted corridors of the hospital.

Two hours later I was 9cm dilated and this baby was

coming. My husband made it just in time as I was whisked into the delivery room. There was no time for any pain relief – everything happened super-fast and I was ready to push. My son, Leo, was born in the early hours. We had skin-to-skin cuddles before he was taken to special care due to being born at 35 weeks. He was healthy though and came home after one week.

I'm so glad that I was strong enough and confident enough to say no to early augmentation. I certainly didn't need anything to be speeded up. I didn't get the calm water birth that I had planned for, but I did have an amazing birth, and I'm proud of what my body achieved.

B is for . . .

BED – GET OFF IT!

During The Happy Birth Club course, the first (and my favourite) exercise we do is this: each couple sketches a picture of the room in which they want to meet their baby. They must picture the scene in detail. Who is there? Is music playing? Is medical equipment on show or in the next room? Is there an epidural or a pool, a Swiss ball or a shower? If it's a **caesarean** birth (see page 115), do they know how many people will be in the room and what music do they want? I ask them to aim high; not to be apologetic if they want fairy lights and champagne on ice in a bucket. You might like to give it a try yourself.

Ninety-nine per cent of the time there is a bed in that drawing. And over 60 per cent will show themselves lying flat on their back on the bed with dad at the head end and midwife or doctor at their feet.

This image is so pervasive that it requires some explanation, and for that we must go back to seventeenth-century France and Louis XIV. Perhaps it was because his mother had four previous stillbirths, or perhaps he was just bit pervy, but Louis demanded that his mistresses gave birth on their backs while he peeped at them from behind a curtain in his Amy Winehouse-style wig. The doctors rather liked this as they didn't have to get their knees dirty by attending to a woman who was usually more upright, closer to the floor. Word got out to the great, squatting masses that the women at court gave birth lying down, and so it became de rigueur: an early precursor of 'too posh to push' – 'too posh to squat'.

Soon after, a French family of male obstetricians called the Chamberlens invented the first medical forceps for pulling babies out. But, crucially, the birthing woman had to be flat on her back on the bed in order for these early doctors to roll up their sleeves and demonstrate their patriarchal prowess.

A lasting effect

Critically, this action signposted a power shift: it's quite hard to feel assertive and in control when you're lying, legs akimbo, frightened and in pain. The subsequent rapid medicalisation and hospitalisation of birth, increased methods of hands-on intervention and more men in the birthing space helped to entrench this practice. Early epidurals required women to be immobilised on a bed. But it soon became normal for all women to lie supine (even without an epidural) and still it remains. Being flat on your back on the bed is easier for doctors and midwives – it is rarely easier for you.

Luckily, we are going back to the future and brand-new NHS birth centres never have a bed in the room. They are often folded up into the wall and brought down once baby is born for you to sleep in. Midwives know that a bed tells women to lie down but they also know it's in your best interests to be upright.

Having said all that, some women prefer to be on the bed giving birth, albeit with the headrest raised and their knees brought upwards to allow the pelvis to be slightly angled downwards, in which case, go with it. Listen to your body and the position in which it feels most comfortable.

Reasons to stay off the bed

- Your pelvis is constricted by 30 per cent when you lie flat. And you never need more pelvic space than when you're breathing out a baby.
- Gravity is your best friend at birth. Babies are generally quite heavy and respond well to the extra help of the Earth's pull. Use it!
- Lying on your back is normally more painful.
- If baby is not in an optimal position (for example, if it is facing backwards) you have very little chance of letting it rotate while on your back.
- Pushing uphill is hard! Imagine lying on your bed to do a poo. Not easy eh?
- You increase your chances of an assisted delivery if you're flat on the bed.
- The baby is getting its oxygen from the cord. Lying flat increases your chances of that being compressed.

- With today's modern, mobile epidurals, you can remain mobile and upright.
- See **positions** (page 274) for alternatives to lying down.

BIRTH BAG

Women tend to get quite agitated about packing a birth bag. I think it may be part of the off-to-war mentality that can beset the days before your due date – especially if you are nervous. You may feel that the one thing you can control is your birth bag and so it's tempting to over-worry about it. Don't. Some women go into labour earlier than expected and manage absolutely fine with hospital gowns, blankets and towels, before sending someone home to get the rest of their gubbins. In the Western world we are never that far from a shop selling nappies.

Getting your bag packed can have that same excitement that comes from preparing for a holiday, however. So if it helps you to get the butterflies going, treat yourself to a few nice things and enjoy!

If you're choosing to give birth in a hospital or birth centre, you'll probably want to have a bag packed and ready to go from about 37 weeks. If you're planning for a straightforward labour, pack for a 24–36 hour stay; however, you might want to prepare a second bag or leave a second pile of extras in case you stay in longer and you can send someone home to get the rest of your stuff. It will prevent potential arguments that begin, 'I didn't mean that cardigan, and where are my knickers?!'

If you're having a home birth, you might still want to pack a bag in case of a transfer to a hospital during labour. This is a suggested list:

- Maternity notes – if you forget these your partner will be sent home for them.
- Birth preference sheet – two copies.
- Baby car seat – fitted. This will avoid standing in the rain reading instructions in a hospital car park.
- Anti-bacterial wipes/spray. If you have a private midwife or doula they will often whizz round the room with these when nobody is looking. Feel free to do the same. Hospital cleaners are busy. They may not have time to match your high standards.
- A change of clothes to go home in – forget the skinny jeans. You'll be in maternity clothes for a few weeks yet – and that's OK. You will probably be a similar size to when you were seven months pregnant.
- Feeding bra – even though your milk doesn't come in for three days, you will produce colostrum. These bras are comfortable, stretchy and give access to your bosoms.
- Partner's clothes. They may want some shorts and T-shirts to wear during labour – hospitals are very hot.
- A change of clothes if you are staying overnight.
- A loo roll. A Happy Birth Club mum told a story of using one of those large plastic loo roll dispensers in the maternity ward. The roll was empty and so she peeked up into the holder to try to grab some paper. The inside edge of the dispenser was covered in dried blood – obviously not a place that was regularly cleaned! This is probably not common. But with this in mind you might want to take your own paper.
- Wash bag, toothbrush, toiletries (for mum and dad). Include fragrance-free shower gel for after the birth.
- Two packets of maternity pads (these are just like sanitary

towels built for heavy flow). You'll need to change them frequently during the first week, but especially during the first 24 hours.

- Several pairs of huge, cheap comfy knickers (stretchy net knickers are popular, but a pack of cheap cotton granny pants are just as good).
- Two loose cottony/button-down shirts/night shirts – you do *not* have to wear hospital gowns (see **gowngate** – page 189).
- Two pairs of cheap pyjama pants (you may leak on them).
- Flip flops that you don't mind wearing in a shower.
- A comfy dressing gown.
- Two pillows in distinctive pillowcases. White ones will go missing. There is a bizarre shortage of pillows on maternity wards. You will love having them to get comfortable before, during and after the birth (and your birth partner might use them for a snooze in the chair).
- Travel hairdryer and brush – you're going to have a lot of photos taken and there won't be a hairdryer lying around. You can thank me later.
- Sports drinks bottle. Ideally filled with ice, as hospitals are very hot and you may not have access to a freezer. If you are moving around during labour or using a pool, it's easier to drink from a sports bottle – your partner can lift it to your mouth without you even having to open your eyes.
- Drinks and snacks for both of you – anything you might fancy to keep your energy up. Birth is a marathon, not a sprint.
- Baby clothes: vest, Babygro, hat. Take three or four complete changes.
- Ten newborn nappies and cotton wool (you may want to

use wipes, but cotton wool and water is a tad kinder to brand-new skin).

- Baby blanket – no cashmere. Hot wash everything you take to hospital to get rid of germs.
- Mobile and charger.
- Massage oil – pure base oil with optional essential oils of your choice.
- **TENS machine** (see page 314), if you fancy using one.
- Fragrance-free lip balm – especially if you use **gas and air** (see page 186) you'll probably find your lips feel dry.
- Flannel – to be used hot or cold in labour.
- Birth ball if you prefer your own or are not sure if your place of birth will supply one.
- Your own mugs – birth should not be followed by tea in a polystyrene cup – you're more important than that. A brew in your own mug will taste like nectar of the gods.

BIRTH CENTRE

Birth centres are midwifery-run units in which you can deliver your baby with minimum medical intervention. There are two types, which are effectively the same except for their location: 'freestanding' and those which are 'alongside' a hospital's labour ward.

In order to understand why birth centres are enjoying a renaissance, have a look at **oxytocin** (see page 257) and **home birth** (see page 197).

Freestanding birth centres are stand-alone units run by midwives containing everything you could need for a natural birth, but in the event of transferring to hospital, you would travel by ambulance. These units generally have outstandingly low rates of intervention, complication or hospital transfer but are becoming increasingly rare as they are often under-used due to a lack of information about them and because the majority of women still feel 'safer' in hospital.

Nevertheless, responding to demand from women for a more homely and less medical environment to labour in and a better understanding of the scientific connection between mind, body and hormones, more hospitals are building or renovating their birth centres. These are known as 'alongside birth centres' and, in most cases, they are situated down the corridor from the delivery suite.

Both types of midwifery-led units are intended to support women who want a natural, drug-free birth but feel that a home birth isn't for them. Many women like the idea of a comfortable, cosy room but feel reassured by the presence of medical backup just along the corridor should they require it.

On your first booking-in appointment, you should be offered a range of options for where to give birth: home birth, birth centre or labour ward. But this does not always happen. If it doesn't – ask!

A more relaxing atmosphere

In a birth centre, the focus is on comfort, freedom of movement, an active birth and a general loveliness that will allow you to tap into your inner goddess, switch off your busy brain and breathe your baby out. All medical equipment that might unnerve you is out of sight but easily accessible should a midwife need it.

Your privacy is respected in birth centres. They pride themselves on woman-centred care and aren't under quite the same time pressures or box-ticking expectations as labour wards. You will commonly be given more time to labour simply because birth centres aren't as busy as the wards. This is mainly because women don't know they exist. Unless you get educated antenatally, it is quite possible to go through an entire pregnancy and labour not knowing that along the corridor from your Victorian hospital room was the birth equivalent of a five-star hotel with fluffy towels.

Birth centres offer pain relief in the form of attentive care: midwives may have hypnosis or aromatherapy/massage skills. They provide birth pools, positioning and also **gas and air** (see page 186). Some units also offer **diamorphine/pethidine** (see page 138), so feel free to ask about your options while on your pre-labour visit. If you need an **epidural** (see page 155) or an **assisted delivery** (see page 53) you will be taken (normally by wheelchair) to the nearby labour ward where there are **obstetricians** (see page 249) and anaesthetists.

Who can use a birth centre?

Each hospital has its own qualification criteria for using its birth centre. This might include maternal age, medical conditions and potential complications that might arise. If you're **induced** (see induction – medical, page 220), for example, you will be prevented from using the birth centre due to increased medical monitoring. But feel free to explore your options fully and discuss your preferences with the hospital.

Fortunately, even delivery suites are cottoning on to the fact that most women feel more relaxed if the environment is less medical and more comfortable. There are also things that you and your partner can do on a labour ward to enhance the levels of comfort.

You will have your own bathroom in the birth centre and can normally stay the night with your partner after delivery.

There can be unhelpful sneering about women who wish to use birth centres – as though they are setting themselves up for disappointment or aiming too high like a crazy birthzilla. But why not have a tour of your local unit and make an informed decision?

BIRTH PLAN

How do you feel about a birth plan?

When I ask this question on my course, people commonly roll their eyes. 'You can't exactly plan a birth, can you?', some say. 'If you write a plan and it goes wrong, you'll be disappointed.'

I say, aim high. Plan away! Yes, things might go differently: sometimes the woman who insists she will have an epidural gets by with a devoted **midwife** and a mere whiff of **gas and air** (see pages 243 and 186); another is sure of wanting a **water birth** (see page 317) but is surprised to find she doesn't fancy the pool at all. Neither of these women will be devastated by the fact that they didn't tick all the boxes on their birth plan. Call me a feminist, but I think women (especially mothers) are bloody strong and resilient – we can cope when plans change.

Having said all that, I do think some women (and men) benefit psychologically from a slightly looser terminology such as a 'birth preference sheet'. This is often more warmly received by some midwives, as it can suggest that you are not so rigid in your mindset that you won't take good medically indicated advice.

Although birth plans, or preference sheets, can get a very bad press in some cases, they are absolutely invaluable; for example, survivors of rape or sexual abuse can feel utterly terrified by the idea of strangers touching their most intimate parts in a brightly lit room. But without a known midwife, that woman is unable to build up such a rapport that she is able to communicate this history.

A written sheet that you can hand over alleviates the need for any awkward or upsetting conversations. It is a brilliant way of having your specific needs met by a kind and caring midwife. Believe me, midwives will want to know such facts so that they can behave in the most considerate manner. But it is not always possible to raise these matters in hurried antenatal visits – and, nevertheless, you might have a different midwife in labour anyway.

A good antenatal course will help you to consider what you might wish to put on your plan. If you would prefer the midwife to listen in to your baby intermittently rather than being strapped to an electronic heartbeat monitoring machine, this is a good place to state that. Discuss your plan with your midwife and factor in any specific requirements: do you have a bad back, which might make certain positions difficult? Your **Hypnobirthing** (see page 206) coach can also be extremely helpful. Ask for their suggestions.

Getting the most from your birth plan

Take three copies to your place of birth and, in the event that there is a shift change, make sure your partner knows to bring out another copy in case the first has gone missing.

Telling the midwife how you have prepared is also important. If you have taken a Hypnobirthing course, she will most likely understand the need to respect your preference for language that doesn't reference 'pain' or 'contractions'. She will also know not to interrupt you with chit-chat unless you begin such interactions.

The sheet opposite is the one I use on the course, but any such layout will do. There are no right or wrong answers. This isn't an exam paper. Every woman's sheet will be different. Take time to consider what is important to you.

BIRTH PREFERENCE SHEET

Hello, my name is ___Jessica Smith_____ and I am __37___ years of age.

This is my __first___ baby. Here are some preferences that I have thought through for my labour. I'm aware of the need to be flexible and I'm happy to work with your suggestions. Please help me to understand any reasons behind decisions that need to be made. My birth companion will help me to listen to your guidance, so please discuss anything with them if I am in my own little world! Many thanks for all that you will do to help us.

Birth companions:
Name(s), relationship and phone number(s):
Chris, husband, 0795562555

How I've prepared for labour:
Antenatal classes, hypnobirthing, yoga.

Induction:

Happy to be induced if medically indicated.
Prefer to start with pessaries and take a slow approach.

Birth pool:

Yes please! I'd love to try the pool but feel – at this stage – that I would prefer to get out for the moment of delivery.

Pain relief:

I will be using hypnobirthing and a TENS machine. Would be open to use of gas and air later in labour. Please don't offer epidural unless I request it.

Movement during labour:

I'd like to remain upright as much as possible and have an active birth – walking, crouching and using the Swiss ball. I'm keen to avoid lying flat on my back on the bed.

Foetal monitoring:

I would prefer intermittent foetal monitoring rather than the electronic version, if that means lying me on the bed. Of course, in the event of an emergency, monitor as necessary.

Internal examinations:

I'd like to avoid these as far as possible. Please can we only do this in the event of needing to make a decision about our next course of action.

Positions to use:

Sitting on the Swiss ball, kneeling, standing, leaning on my partner.

Perineum:

Please protect my perineum as much as possible. I wish to avoid an episiotomy.

Caesarean birth:

If this occurs as an emergency situation, please help me to have skin-to-skin contact with my baby as soon as possible.

Meeting baby:

I would like you to catch my baby and bring him (or her) up to my chest as soon as possible. Please allow my husband to tell me the sex.

Placenta, or third stage:

If we have had a drug-free birth, I would like to have a physiological third stage with natural delivery of the placenta.

Vitamin K and immunisations:

I would prefer my baby to receive vitamin K orally, rather than via injection – thanks.

Other stuff I'd feel happier if you knew:

I have a terrible fear of needles! So please support me to have my baby without an epidural as far as possible. If we do go to theatre for a C-section, please inform the anaesthetist of my phobia and help distract me. Thank you for helping me to meet my baby!

BLOOD

Along with the idea that birth is to be feared, sits the myth that it is also so gory that it wouldn't look out of place in a Quentin Tarantino film. The truth is, it's not.

Yes, there will be a little bit of blood for the midwife to deal with – how much varies from woman to woman – but you will be so busy looking at your beautiful new baby that you will barely notice it.

In a birth pool it can look like a lot, so don't be scared if you have a **water birth** (see page 317) and look down to see what appears to be a scene from *Jaws*. Just like a drop of blood in a sink of water, it will appear magnified.

Bleeding during pregnancy is one of the very few red lights that can indicate a serious problem. Any sign of this mustn't be ignored, especially if you have a low-lying placenta. Any sign of blood should be taken seriously and you will need to make contact with your **midwife** (see page 243) or maternity unit.

It is difficult to know which women will bleed significantly during labour and which will not – although the type of birth you have may make a difference. If you tear or have an **episiotomy** (see page 161) during delivery, then your bleeding can be increased, but it won't concern you at that stage as you gaze lovingly at your babba.

If you are bleeding too much after the birth, the care providers will work swiftly to make sure that it does not become more serious. Any large amounts of blood loss would be considered the sign of a post-partum haemorrhage, and this happens in only about 5 per cent of births. Some women will be compromised by this, others won't. It's a very individual experience. It is not an exact science, but one woman would feel fine after losing as much as 750ml, whereas another women would feel faint and tired after losing 300ml (which is not classified as a post-partum haemorrhage, as this is 500ml).

The placenta is definitely the goriest bit of birth and you can choose to look – or look away – as it is delivered. Men tend to find it quite fascinating. The placenta is a wonderful, life-giving organ that we should probably worship. It's nothing to be feared, so take a look if you want to (although you may never order steak tartare for lunch again – just saying). At home births the midwives will efficiently dispose of the placenta. If you have older children, let them have a look at it before it is taken away. That's one biology lesson that their schoolmates will never enjoy! The placenta is the source of all life, and children are commonly less squeamish than us – in fact, boys seem to love the goriness of a fresh placenta.

BRAXTON HICKS

This might sound like the name of an author of dystopian fiction, but it was in fact an English doctor, John Braxton Hicks, who – in 1872 – spent his time investigating pregnancy and discovered that mild, tightening contractions occur towards the end of gestation but before labour. One hundred and forty-four years later, his name is still uttered across the world when women pause for breath and place a hand on their bump as they attentively consider if this sensation is 'it'.

You may not even notice these tightenings, so they are nothing to worry about. It's basically your uterus contracting and relaxing throughout pregnancy – a sort of toning exercise going on inside for your benefit. Don't feel silly if you mistake them for actual labour – many, many women do. Labour contractions tend to start short and sharpish. Braxton Hicks close to your due date may last two minutes at a time so that is a good way of differentiating between the two. But if in doubt, let your midwife know.

BREASTFEEDING

If you think birth is a sensitive issue, just wait until you hop on the milk-train. This is where you buy a ticket to the emotional highs and lows that set you up quite nicely for a lifetime of parenting.

Regardless of how you might feel at this very moment, all fecund and fabulous, it's oddly impossible to know how you will view breastfeeding until your baby arrives. I know women who swore they'd never do it, still offering up their nipple to a six-year-old at a tea party and those, convinced it would be a doddle, shocked to find it was a lonely, painful, dispiriting time that they flashback to at the mere sight of a cherry bun.

Successful breastfeeding is free, convenient, rewarding and joyful. And any breastfeeding is good breastfeeding. But it doesn't always come naturally. There are many personal, economic, emotional and cultural reasons why women don't breastfeed. But often it's because there is nobody around to help them emotionally or practically in the first weeks.

The UK has the lowest breastfeeding rate in the world. Our figures have fallen in line with the number of hours bestowed on caring for women postnatally – by either the NHS or simply by the demise of close-knit communities in which women of all generations rallied round a new mum. Before you leave your place of birth, a **midwife** (see page 243) should watch you complete a full breastfeed from start to finish. Midwives might laugh at the suggestion that they would have time for that 'luxury', but if you aren't satisfied, speak to the supervisor of midwives until you are. Today, women are sent home after 24 hours with a brief midwife visit booked for the following day. Consequently, far too many women are struggling alone. It's a horrible, guilt-inducing combination of factors: women are given leaflets telling them that they must breastfeed, but are then sent home to suffer in silence. This is the worst possible combination resulting in thousands of very unhappy new mummies.

Working on busy wards, midwives frequently feel under pressure to prematurely offer formula to new mums. Almost 100 per cent of the women on our course who use one particular hospital are given formula within the first 24 hours because they 'aren't producing enough milk'.

As feeding is a difficult balancing act with your boobs producing their supply based on your baby's demands, using a bottle within the first 48 hours can seriously derail your breastfeeding plans. Brand new babies need nothing more than the teeny amount of colostrum that you provide immediately after birth.

Watch out for the unhelpful reactions

Remember that health professionals are human too – they will have their own baggage, preconceptions and possible prejudices. Most of them will be kind and knowledgeable. But not all know exactly what they're talking about. Under 'bollocks about breast-feeding' I've heard women told by 'experts' that their 'nipples are the wrong shape', their boobs are 'dry' (even though they gave birth 12 hours earlier and their milk won't come in for another two or three days) and, my personal favourite, 'your baby just doesn't want to breastfeed'. That's right, a newborn baby that was clearly looking for a chai latte rather than its mother's bosom.

Like a happy birth experience, successful breastfeeding isn't a matter of luck. If you don't get support and suddenly find yourself swimming in a sea of viciously conflicting emotions, reaching for a safe place while the only rocks available are strapped to your chest and on fire, then this is not a happy place. I want you to be happy and able to enjoy your baby.

Question everything! Return to this book, seek qualified, local, recommended, hands-on support and consider booking a private midwife or lactation consultant who will visit you at home and take time to show you where things might be going wrong. It may be as simple as positioning your baby on the boob, or perhaps you will be prescribed pasta bakes and litres of water while wallowing in bed for some serious skin-to-skin action to get the hormones (and thus milk) flowing.

The benefits of getting the right help

I fed my own babies for about three to five months (a little less with each child – which is pretty typical due to the demands made by the other children). It can be tiring, and the responsibility of keeping a human alive on your milk alone can feel immense. But the health benefits for me and baby outweighed the potential pitfalls. My mum had fed me and my siblings; I had confidence that it would be possible. But there is no way I could have breastfed without Pam's hands-on support in the first few days after my milk came in. It would have been too physically agonising and I would definitely have given a bottle of formula between wiping the tears of pain from my eyes. I would have felt guilty and felt like a failure, as I believed breastfeeding was best for my baby and I wanted to do it. I despair at the numbers of women who find themselves in this position without good help and advice. I had my own mum as well as Pam to encourage me and teach me. It got easier and then, overall, it was convenience that kept me going.

Less than 1 per cent of women are incapable of breastfeeding for physiological reasons. So, with that in mind, consider the pros and cons of breastfeeding and start thinking about it before your baby arrives – this is my exhaustive list.

The advantages of breastfeeding

- It's free, leaving you more to spend on much-needed lattes with your new mummy friends.

- It kick-starts your baby's immune system: it protects against infections and diseases.
- It significantly lessens the chances of allergies including asthma and eczema.
- It's on tap – the convenience of feeding in a car park on a rainy day when you're running late cannot be overstated.
- It's the right temperature: no waiting for a bottle to warm/ cool with a screaming baby.
- It's a great excuse to sit down. Nobody can expect you to empty the dishwasher or cook dinner while you're feeding. Do not look this gift horse in the mouth. Never again will you have such a great excuse to sit down with the TV remote control, a good book or simply your baby's beautiful face to gaze at. (Sometimes, I wish I had carried on feeding my kids into their school years just so that I could occasionally sit down.)
- Once breastfeeding is successfully established, night feeds are quicker and easier than preparing formula.
- The face of a satisfied baby, drunk on milk, will be one of the sights that gets you through those hard days and nights.
- Your baby is less likely to be hospitalised with vomiting and diarrhoea because their immunity is better and they haven't absorbed bacteria or had a reaction to formula.
- Your baby is less likely to be obese as an older child. Although this is a much more complicated issue, it's true that breastfed babies will 'pop off' the boob when full. It's impossible to overfeed a breastfed baby. The theory is that in developing this satisfied reflex, children learn to recognise this same feeling when toddlers, infants and, eventually, teenagers.
- It is a great way to settle a fractious baby ('fractious' is a

word that you will never have used but will hear every day from the moment they are born).

- Nappies smell quite pleasant when baby is fed on breast milk alone.
- It significantly reduces your chances of breast and ovarian cancer.
- It burns up to 500 calories a day! Whoop, whoop!
- It tightens your knackered uterus so that your bleeding stops sooner and your tummy flattens sooner. Whoop, whoop!
- Breastfed babies do better at 11-plus exams. This is a fact. But really, do we think this is because they were breastfed? I think not.

The challenges of breastfeeding

- You can't weed the garden, go for a run or paint the hallway while you are sitting down breastfeeding. It stops you doing stuff you really want to get done. This is Mother Nature's way of getting us to slow down, but I believe this is one of the biggest barriers for modern women who feel we need to be 'productive' at all times. It demands a shift in our mindset.
- You can feel that you aren't making enough milk. This might be true, but your low supply may be because you are running around and not eating/drinking enough (see above). If this is the case, be honest with yourself and others. It's important to understand, recognise and accept this so that you can choose whether to slow down and prioritise breastfeeding or keep yourself happy, stimulated and fulfilled by switching to formula.
- The first two to three days after your milk comes in can be incredibly painful for some women. If you don't have

the right emotional and practical support, giving up will feel like a good idea.

- It's not as easy to go away for a night/weekend without your baby unless you want to do a lot of expressing to keep your supply flowing or ease the discomfort of full boobs. Again, this is a personal choice. We live a life of endless options. No previous generation had to consider their priorities in parenthood as much as we do.

- You need to eat and drink lots to keep your milk supply plentiful. It's easy to forget to do so when you are so busy with a new baby.

- It might make your boobs a bit more saggy (but pregnancy alone has done its work there). Exercise and good bras will help.

- Sore nipples – is almost always a problem of position. If your baby is not latched on properly it will be sucking on the delicate sticky-out bit of your nipple, and this can quickly cause the skin to split and bleed. (See midwife Chloe's advice below regarding latch).

- But even with a good latch, it is normal to feel some discomfort as the milk rushes down to your nipple once baby is attached. This can really sting, but it should only last a few seconds, so breathe deeply, drop your shoulders and wait a few moments for the sensation to recede. If the baby is sucking in a great position, the pain will rather magically fade away. This let-down feeling normally only lasts a few days rather than weeks, and eventually it will feel less painful and more like a satisfying fullness: a handy cue that your milk is plentiful.

- Wet boobs – if you're a leaker (and not everyone is), you'll go through lots of breast pads. It's just something else to carry in your bulging nappy bag, and once feeding is well established you'll probably dispense with the pads altogether.

- At first, you will need a good memory – which breast did I feed from last? Use an app or go old school and use a safety pin on your bra strap or a bracelet on your wrist to remind you which boob you fed from last. It might help to keep a little diary to hand, especially after the first three to four weeks when you might be trying to find a little routine. Eventually, you will instinctively know which breast you fed from last, as it will be the empty one.
- You might not like the feel of it.
- Partners – some men think the boobs belong to them. These men are idiots. Some men – who are genuinely trying to be helpful – urge the use of formula.
- You might not feel especially sexy while breastfeeding. If you want to get back in the saddle sooner, this might be an incentive to stop.
- You may feel self-conscious feeding in public. Although I'd rather you got your knockers out with complete abandon everywhere from Claridge's Tearoom to your local swimming pool, in a culture that sexualises boobs on the pages of national newspapers, it's very common to feel embarrassed about such exposure.
- If *you* feel better covering up a little with a muslin cloth over your shoulder, then go for it (you may also need such a cover if you're feeding in the summer and have to protect your baby from the sun). But once you've got the hang of feeding, you will probably find that any initial embarrassment makes way for a devil-may-care attitude until one day you realise you're in Starbucks with both bosoms out while discussing the consistency of baby poo. Or, once you get skilled at feeding, you will find that

you can do so without exposing any more skin than you would in an average V-necked T-shirt.

- Feeding can be a fashion nightmare. You'll need bras with clips and tops that can be unbuttoned or lifted to the side. Goodbye polo necks, hello cardigans.
- It's harder to know if your baby has had enough, and some personality types find this impossible.

How do I get started?

Crucially, get your baby on the breast as quickly as you can after birth. Your midwife should encourage this unless you have specifically requested that you don't want this.

Your new baby's tummy is absolutely tiny – it can only hold about 8ml of fluid. It needs to feed little and often; not have its stomach stretched by 30ml of formula!

You will only produce colostrum at the start – you may never even see it except in the form of baby poo. It is yellow in colour and packed full of antibodies, nutrients and vitamins. Your boobs will produce roughly 5ml of this for each feed – which is perfect.

After two, three or sometimes four days, your baby may be noticeably unsettled and fractious. Don't panic and reach for the formula. This is their way of telling your body that they are growing, their tummy is expanding and that they are about to need more milk. Human bodies are simply amazing.

What happens next?

Depending on your hormone production, you may suddenly experience the sort of immediate boob job that a porn queen could only dream about. This can coincide with a drop in happy hormones – so you get mahoosive sore bazookas and a type of temporary tearfulness – another of Mother Nature's little jokes.

This is the most testing time for new mums, and it is so easy to give up at this point. It can be very painful to feed now – even with a good latch.

If your boobs are hugely engorged, it might be impossible for your baby to latch on. Don't be tempted to reach for the pump, as you will simply be telling your body to fill dem bad boys all the way up again. You may just need to release a bit of milk so that the area around your nipple softens and baby can get a good mouthful.

Instead of pumping at this stage, try these alternatives:

- Hand express in a *hot* bath – as hot as you can stand. Lean forward, make a fist with your right hand and massage down the right breast from the top, under the armpit all the way to the nipple. Use a little soap on your skin if you prefer. Be patient. It can take a while and might hurt like hell. The heat will draw out some milk and you should see it emerge into the water. Just let it flow. It isn't wasted milk. You need to ease the engorgement and soften the skin around your nipple so that the baby can latch on. The pain will be worth it when you get out, with softer, less heavy boobs. You should only really need to do this once or twice in the first 24–72 hours after your milk has come in. After that, your body should have found its own rhythm.
- While feeding, massage your boob towards the nipple from under the armpit. This should encourage the milk to come down.
- If you're in a lot of pain, take a mild pain reliever such as paracetamol or ibuprofen.

- Engorged breasts that don't empty can cause plugged ducts (sore, hard lumps in your breast tissue). This can lead to mastitis – milk that has become infected inside the breast. This can be extremely painful and may require antibiotics. Contact your midwife, health visitor or GP for advice, especially if you develop a temperature.
- If your baby is latching on well and your milk is letting down efficiently, your silicone-like footballs should soften and calm down after two or three days

How often should I feed my baby?

Breast milk is capitalist – it works strictly on a *supply-and-demand* basis. If you need more milk you need to keep baby on longer and more regularly. If you don't ask anything of your breasts, they won't give you anything. You can't overfeed a breastfed baby. Watch their cues and, if in doubt, bring them to the breast. Forget the idea of a feeding routine until at least four to six weeks when things may settle down a little. In the first two to three weeks, it is more important to keep your milk supply flowing by letting your boobs know you have a baby to feed. The more baby nurses, the more milk you will make. But if the latch is not correct, prolonged feeding will lead to very sore nipples, so it will be hurting for minutes rather than seconds – get advice.

What do I need to buy?

Almost nothing. That's the beauty of breastfeeding; however, you may find these help the practicalities:

- **Breast pads** (disposable or recyclable) For most women these will be essential, especially in the first few weeks or months. But if you find you are not a leaker, you may never need them.

- **Breastfeeding bra** Three or four good breastfeeding bras will give optimal comfort, reduce the risk of blocked ducts and make breastfeeding more simple. They will get sweaty and milky and will be in and out of the washing machine. You won't know what size you need until your milk supply is established (and your back may narrow quite noticeably within the first three weeks after you've given birth). Start with the bra that fits you at the end of your pregnancy and treat yourself to some new ones once baby has arrived.

- **Breastfeeding pillow** A good breastfeeding pillow is not essential, but can be very handy in the early days while getting to grips with positioning and attachment. Alternatively, regular pillows can be used, and eventually life will be easier if you can feed without any pillow.

- **Muslins** You can never have too many of these. Place one over your shoulder to catch any milky burps when winding between feeds and to protect your clothes.

- **Nipple cream** Not every woman will find that she needs nipple cream to keep the skin soft, but as it is so delicate a little moisturising can help protect the skin and has no negative side effects. Use cream sparingly.

- **Sports bottle of water** to keep with you on the sofa or by the bed in easy reach. Breastfeeding will fill you with the most unimaginable thirst, especially at the moment of letting down. Be prepared for this and keep your supply up by drinking litres of water.

- **Vacuum flask/mug** It's hard to imagine that a hot cup of tea will one day be a luxury item, but it's true, so invest in a good heat-retaining mug with a lid so that your brew remains warm even when you've had its consumption interrupted 27 times in two hours.

- **Food** You need to eat well, plenty and often, to keep your milk supply up. Nurture yourself with nutritious home-cooked meals (they don't need to be cooked by you) and don't even think about dieting.

Expressing/pumping

One of the wonderful things about dads being more involved in childcare is that they can give you an occasional break from feeding. One of the difficult things about dads being involved in childcare is that they can give you an occasional break from feeding. What I mean is that although delegating the odd feed is extremely liberating, if you want to breastfeed, you must wait at least two to three weeks until your supply is completely established and your feeding is going well before you start expressing and offering bottles. Some lactation consultants would even argue that four to six weeks is a safer option if you want to carry on breastfeeding.

This is because an electric or handheld pump is a more intense means of drawing milk from your boobs, messing about with the supply-and-demand process. Also, a bottle is much easier to suck from – just tipping it upside down you will see some droplets. So your baby doesn't have to work as hard to suck. They're learning to feed, of course, so messing around with their wonderful new toy can cause nipple confusion – you might find that you put them on the boob and they don't suck as hard. It really is a delicate business to get the feeding established so, as lovely as it is to have a keen partner, keep them on nappy, winding and walking duty for as long as you can.

Having said that, expressing is a godsend if you want to maintain breastfeeding while also gaining a little freedom. With more and more women returning to work but wanting to keep their supply going, pumping, for them, can become a way of life. Even if you just want a date-night trip to the cinema, knowing you can leave the babysitter with a bottle of expressed milk can be a huge weight off your mind.

You will need a breast pump, but wait before purchasing one, as they're expensive and you might not need one right away (or at all). If you are expressing regularly, it may be beneficial to hire or buy a more powerful one. For normal pumping, an electric or battery-powered one is generally best.

When is the best time to give the pumped feed?

The temptation will be for dad to do the 3am feed so that you can sleep through, but it's important to feed during the night when your prolactin hormone levels are at their highest. If you drop this feed, don't be surprised if your supply soon falls throughout the day.

As long as you are still feeding during the night, the best time to express is probably first thing in the morning. This is when you will probably find your supply is the most plentiful, as you've done little else but lie down for the last eight hours or so, waking only to feed and change your baby. Place your baby on one breast and completely empty it. Then – at the same time or just after – use the other breast to express from. Remember, you will have to sterilise the pump attachments and the bottle that you are filling, or it will be unusable.

Pumping will probably feel very weird, and you won't believe your eyes the first time you see milk squirting out of the tiny holes in your nipples. The machines are pretty noisy and, sadly, sound rather like a cow mooing in a milking shed, giving the whole exercise an unfortunate bovine air. You might struggle to produce much milk, as you need **oxytocin** (see page 257) to get the milk coming down and, without your baby's soft skin making you go all gooey, this might be difficult. Women who pump at work often say that they need to look at a picture of their baby while doing so, as it helps them relax and produce the right love chemicals. It's weird but true.

You will also need something to store expressed breast milk in. For freezing, you could use a sterile ice container with a lid for small amounts of milk, or use milk freezer bags. These are good options and prevent wastage, as you can defrost small or large quantities depending upon your needs.

This means that you are starting the day with no milk in your boobs, so have a good breakfast, drink plenty and don't rush out to the shops. Potter around the house or, even better, stay in bed watching TV with your little snuffle monster and wait for your boobs to fill up again ready for the mid-morning feed. It sounds complicated and it does take some forward planning, but if you can breastfeed and express, you're doing brilliantly and will be able to buy yourself some time away from your baby, if that's what you need.

If you don't want to express – thereby delegating a feed to your partner – because you really enjoy it and view it as a privilege, try to discuss this sensitively. If you're raising a child together, you have many, many years ahead of shared care. It's OK for a new mum to want to hunker down and love her little bundle to pieces.

The Happy Birth Club breastfeeding expert is Chloe Dymond Tucker (RM LFHom IBCLC), a lovely midwife with experience at King's College Hospital, Guy's and St Thomas', plus a year in a Balinese birth centre. She is a fully qualified lactation consultant who works as an NHS community breastfeeding lead in Lambeth, seeing up to 70 women per week. This is her perspective:

Chloe Dymond Tucker on breastfeeding

Everyone says breastfeeding is difficult – is it?

This is most women's number-one fear. Although it's not a walk in the park, the majority of women who are committed to the job reap the benefits that breastfeeding brings. For some women it establishes easily, although the first week is always a steep learning curve for any mother.

Remember, you've just given birth, you have a new baby that you've met for the first time, your body is recovering from pregnancy, your hormones are rebalancing and you're embarking on the journey of motherhood, which is a whole new career you've had little training for. Your sole responsibility at this time is to feed your baby and keep it alive.

Even if breastfeeding does not come easily, with the right early support and a positive attitude, you will be well on the way to being a breastfeeding pro. Understand a little about the physiology and anatomy as well as some basic theory of positioning and attachment.

What can I do to prepare for breastfeeding before I give birth?

Watch a few breastfeeding videos online or download the NHS app Baby Buddy. I'd also recommend learning how to hand express, as this comes in handy during the early days while encouraging baby to latch or collecting the early milk for baby if you need more practice with the latch. It is now a requirement in the NHS that all pregnant women should be taught hand expressing antenatally as well as postnatally, so if you haven't been shown, ask your midwife. You can practise this skill from 37 weeks pregnant and you might even see the colostrum (early milk) before your baby has been born.

What role can my partner play?

Make sure you attend a good breastfeeding session with your partner during your pregnancy. Most partners who take paternity leave end up playing a major role in establishing breastfeeding. They time the feeds, change the nappies, check the latch from all angles and are excellent at calming a fraught baby that is struggling to latch. Partners are frequently described as the woman's rock to survival, and so they'll feel a whole lot more useful if they have an idea of how they can help from the word go.

My partner doesn't want me to feed but I want to – what can I tell them?

There are a number of reasons your partner might not want you to breastfeed, as mentioned earlier. They may feel left out or rejected as the new mother and baby bond through breastfeeding. Some partners want to help by giving a bottle and feel they can't do this if the baby is breastfed. On a superficial level, concerns that breastfeeding cause saggy boobs or affects the figure could be underlying reasons. Some partners see breastfeeding as a struggle and strain on the new mother. They may have experienced a previous breastfeeding scenario that negatively affected someone they cared for.

With these things in mind, be sensitive to their

concerns. Talk about the reasons why they don't want you to breastfeed. Explain how important it is to you and the benefits – show them this book. Suggest you go to the breastfeeding session together so that they have an opportunity to learn more and ask questions. As a parent, your partner is going to want what's best for their baby, so explaining the benefits of breastfeeding can help make them feel it is the right choice, even if they may have to make some sacrifices; however, most of the concerns are illusions and can be quickly turned into positives. Here are some suggestions as to how the partner can be involved with the breastfeeding process:

- Help time the feeds in the early days and remember which breast to feed from. You should aim to empty one breast at each feed and you may struggle to remember which one you used last. By timing the feeds you will be able to better assess if your baby's cries are due to hunger or tiredness.
- Help calm a crying baby with skin-to-skin and rocking or walking.
- Bring food and water for the mother.
- Help check the position and latch – or hold the smartphone so that mum can watch.
- Once breastfeeding is established, the mother can express a feed for the partner to give from a bottle if they want to do this. Frequently this would happen in the evening to give the woman a break.

Isn't formula milk just as good?
In simple terms *no*! Artificial milk is what it says on the packet: 'artificial': man-made and derived from

predominantly cow's milk. Of course, it is a reasonable substitute and it has improved in quality over the years, but it does not match the benefits of human breast milk fed to a baby by its mother. Human milk is perfectly composited to meet the needs of your individual baby. It is totally unique and supports still-developing organs and systems.

How important is early support and where can I find it?

Crucial! This could be from your midwife or a breastfeeding specialist. Get them to check the positioning and attachment, giving support and feedback. Finally, try to keep an open mind. Other mother's experiences can be very different from your own, so just take it all in your stride. Remember, it's your baby, and your happiness is the most important factor, so make sure it's you that makes the decisions about whether breastfeeding is going well or is even achievable for you.

Getting support with breastfeeding is essential, especially in the early days. It's the difference between a smooth and a rough ride. Note that you will get an overload of advice from many different people, ranging from midwives, family, health visitors and even grannies in the street! Much of it may be conflicting and confusing, so ensure you get a midwife to watch a feed before leaving the hospital, and ask for their advice during your community visits. You may need a little more than this though.

If you need more help, websites such as: Le Leche League, Best Beginnings and The Breastfeeding Network will all have reliable information. American

sites such as Kelly Mom and Jack Newman may also
be good resources if you come across problems. There
are breastfeeding helplines, such as the Breastfeeding
Network, where you can get telephone support. Many
communities have breastfeeding cafés where you can go
and get free support once you've been discharged home
from hospital. Make sure you get this information before
leaving the hospital. Many children centres will have
breastfeeding experts in the form of midwives, health
visitors and lactation consultants where you can get
specialist help and meet other breastfeeding mothers.
Antenatal groups may also provide breastfeeding
support.

If you come across a more complex problem, you may
require a lactation consultant. Ensure you hire a reputable
one (ideally recommended by someone you trust) and
try to stick with one person you trust and believe in,
otherwise you may end up very confused.

How should I hold my baby to feed?
Always have baby facing you – if your baby's body is
facing away from your breast, they will have to turn their
head to feed. As you can imagine, this is not comfy for
baby, doesn't make it easy for them to swallow and creates
a poor seal, which could affect the latch, and they might
take in air, making them windy.

Support your baby along the spine and around the
shoulder girdle and bottom of the head. This might
change slightly as baby gets bigger and has better head
control; however, a newborn baby will need good support
and head guidance. Never put your hand on the back of
your baby's head as it restricts them from coming off when

they're done. Check out pictures and videos, and practise with a doll while your pregnant.

Always aim your baby's nose at the nipple – most women don't have to touch their breast at all. They should be looking at where the breast naturally lies and bringing the baby to the breast, rather than the breast to the baby. Wait for a wide mouth from baby and then scoop baby onto the breast. Hold baby securely and closely until they have a good latch and have started to suck rhythmically.

Baby should have their nose free at the top and chin nuzzled into the breast. The dark part of the areola should be seen above baby's nose and the cheeks should look rounded. Little movements in the baby's ear can be seen during sucking, and sucks should be observed followed by a swallow.

What is the 'latch' and why is it important?
The latch is a word you'll hear a lot once you've started breastfeeding. This refers to the way that the baby attaches to the breast. You probably think that as long as it's attached what's the problem? I cannot overstate how important a good latch is – it is the key to successful breastfeeding. A poor latch can cause all kinds of issues. Some babies are able to latch to the breast very easily and can adjust themselves in order to have a perfect feed each time. If this is the case, you are very lucky. It is more likely that you will have to work on the latch for the first week or so in order to perfect it. Remember, you are new to this and so is your newborn baby. Everyone is different and there are many variables to the equation.

Ideally, your nipple (the bit that sticks out) should be

only the top half of what's in your baby's mouth and beneath that should be the whole underside of your areola – the dark circle around your nipple.

Your baby should be facing you and supported along the back and shoulder girdle with your opposite arm to the breast you're feeding from. Remember, your baby has little control over their head so you need to support and guide your baby's head towards the breast with confidence. Start by tickling the nipple on your baby's nose and wait for her to tilt her head back and stick out her tongue, opening her mouth as wide as she can and reaching around like a little sparrow. This is the part where you swiftly move her head towards your breast, chin first. You want her tongue to scoop the underside of the areola with the chin pressed against the breast. Her tongue draws the breast into the mouth and her top lip hooks over the nipple. Bring her in closely and hold her there so that she can draw the nipple towards her soft palate where it will sit.

A strong seal is made creating a negative pressure. Movement from her jaw massages the underside of the breast, pushing milk through the straw-like ducts, out of the nipple and into the back of baby's mouth. The latch should be comfortable. It should feel as though your baby is drawing the breast in with each suck. It may be sore to begin with as your nipples haven't been through this amount of sucking action before and these babies have a strong suction.

If you feel that your baby is biting or pinching at the nipple, then the latch is not quite right. Use a little finger to break the seal between your baby's cheek and your breast. Start again. A shallow latch could lead to cracked, painful nipples. Not having enough breast in your baby's mouth could prevent baby from draining all the milk from your breasts. This could lead to baby's weight gain being slow; prolonged, frequent feeds; an unsettled colicky baby, as well as blocked ducts, engorgement or even mastitis for the mother.

Most of the time, a little practice and support will ensure that a mother and her baby can perfect the art of a good latch. There are occasionally reasons why babies are unable to achieve a proper latch, most commonly is if your baby has a tongue-tie.

What is a tongue-tie?
Tongue-tie is when the frenulum (the piece of skin attaching the tongue to the base of the mouth) is short and tight. This restricts movement of the tongue and can affect the latch.

Midwives (see page 243) should check for a tongue-tie before you leave the hospital/birth centre, but they often go undetected.

In some babies, the tie is obvious and the tongue even appears forked at the tip, whereas in others, the tongue appears normal to the untrained eye. If you find your baby is getting frustrated on the boob; failing to gain weight or making a clicking sound when feeding, ask an expert for their opinion. Trust your instinct. A very simple procedure to painlessly snip the tie can transform your breastfeeding experience. But bear in mind that on the NHS you may have to wait two to three weeks to get this procedure done, by which time you may have had to give up breastfeeding. Make a fuss and beg to be seen as soon as possible.

Private lactation specialists will normally come to your home to carry out the procedure for about £100. Tongue-ties tend not to affect bottle feeding, as this demands much less of the baby in terms of sucking effort.

What is the difference between hind milk and fore milk?

Once your milk has come in, your baby is likely to get a full meal from just one breast. This isn't always the case, as it depends on the capacity of milk each breast holds and sometimes your baby may want a little extra, but one breast per feed is the norm.

A full breast of milk will contain all the nutrients your baby needs for healthy growth, as well as a high percentage of water for appropriate hydration. Your milk has a very high percentage of lactose as well as a concentration of proteins and fats. The first part of the baby's feed is the fore milk – it has a high concentration of water and lactose, helping to hydrate baby and fill her tummy. This is like the first course of a meal. This milk tends to come out easily as the let-down reflex ejects the milk forcefully and plentifully into baby's mouth. You can hear and see baby gulping and guzzling at this stage. Some babies may pull back if the let down is fast and the milk is coming out more quickly than they can swallow.

Once the feed settles in, you'll notice baby sucking rhythmically using big jaw movements to draw the milk in. Towards the end of the feed, the milk ejection slows down. The baby has to work harder to get the milk out. This milk is much more concentrated, with a higher percentage of fat. It is thicker and more calorific and is called the hind milk. It is fattier and more concentrated than the fore milk. This part of the feed fills up the baby and helps with weight gain.

How will I know if my baby is/isn't getting enough?
If a baby is not latched to the breast well, it may not be able to get this hind milk out efficiently. They will stay at the breast for over an hour and ask for feeds more frequently. The baby may appear unsettled, not put on sufficient weight or start having green poos instead of yellow ones. Mothers may find their milk supply reduces or they end up with blocked ducts as the thick fatty milk sits in the ducts, becoming sticky and affecting flow. Blocked ducts can become inflamed, which may lead to mastitis. If you have any concerns over the latch it is wise to seek assistance sooner rather than later. Observe your baby and their feeds.

Are they:

- Putting on sufficient weight?
- Doing one to two yellow poos a day? (Note that some baby's do poo less, so check everything else is OK if that's the case.)
- Producing six to eight wet nappies per day?
- Having two- to three-hour gaps between feeding?
- Looking satisfied after most feeds?
- Having feeds that mainly last under one hour? (Some babies cluster feed for hours at a time in the evenings though – this is OK.)
- Looking healthy?
- Feeding enough to make your breasts soft and comfortable?

Remember that it is normal for your baby to lose weight in the first week – about 5 per cent of their birth weight as they've passed all the heavy meconium that was in their tummies at birth. After that most babies gain 140–200g per week.

What if I don't make enough milk?

This is a common fear among breastfeeding mothers. It tends to be the main reason women give for stopping breastfeeding. Mothers will tell this tale to other women and the worry kicks in long before the pregnant woman has even given birth. Please remember that we've survived and evolved for centuries on breast milk. You can and will make enough milk as long as you understand the mechanism of your milk supply: you rest, eat and drink plenty of water and take your time to feed.

If your milk supply reduces, there are always solutions to increase it again. Less than 1 per cent of women are unable to produce enough milk, and this is usually down to a medical reason, such as breast reduction, thyroid problem or hyperplasia (a lack of breast tissue). Yet even women with these conditions can often produce enough milk, but they may need extra support.

An inefficient latch might affect how well the breast is stimulated, which is why the latch is important. There is much help you can get if this is the problem.

Remember, your breast-milk supply is based on how much you demand, so introducing bottles of formula will tell your body to make less milk.

Put your baby to the breast more frequently to build

up your supply. Some women find that using a pump a couple of times a day will also help to up the quantity of milk.

Do you have any top tips for sitting comfortably?
Holding your baby in a comfy position during feeds is one of the most important factors to successful breastfeeding as well as ensuring an efficient latch, so the two will go hand in hand. The position you feed in will depend on your anatomy, shape and size as well as your baby's anatomy and size. There's no exact science, which is why some mothers and babies need a little extra support adopting a position that's right for them.

You do not necessarily need to buy a specific feeding pillow, but some women swear by them. I like My Brest Friend pillows, as they have a firm base and clip around the mother. It gives relief to the arms and can help with the under-arm hold. You could also try with one or two standard pillows. Women with larger breasts might find that rolling a muslin up and placing it under the breast helps with the lift.

Try to sit up relatively straight and keep your shoulders relaxed (ask your partner to point out if your shoulders are up around your ears).

Get organised before you start, with your drink and perhaps your phone, a good book or remote control. Also, keep your changing bag nearby so that you can change your baby mid-feed, if necessary, without too much effort.

How long should I breastfeed for?

You can breastfeed for as long as you like. The World Health Organization (WHO) recommends breastfeeding up until two years of age. Your baby will start taking solid food from six months, although they may not take much to begin with. By one year old, you can start giving babies cow's milk, and your baby is likely to be eating regular solid meals; however, many babies will still take regular breastfeeds and do still need milk as part of their diets. Many women stop breastfeeding when they have to return to work, although it is possible to express and also to feed baby before and after work. There are rights to breastfeeding and expressing in the workplace, which are worth looking into if this is your plan. The choice is individual to you as a mum. Some women envisage stopping at six months, but then enjoy it so much that they decide to continue for longer.

Some babies wean themselves off the breast, in which case the mother finds a natural end to breastfeeding with that baby. Your baby will always benefit from getting your breast milk, so as long as you're happy and able, it is going to give your child a great start to life. Some women continue to breastfeed beyond the two years, and that's OK as well, as long as it fits in with your lifestyle.

How easy is to stop breastfeeding once I've started?

This is not a straightforward answer. It depends on when you want to stop and why. It depends on your baby and also on you. Physiologically stopping the breast milk shouldn't be too hard. Psychologically stopping might be more of a problem for both mother and baby. If you've decided, for whatever reason, that you just don't want to breastfeed any more, then there are a couple of methods to stop milk production. First, you could just stop! You will probably be uncomfortable for a few days. Use cold compresses on engorged breasts and, if necessary, massage a little milk out in a hot shower to relieve the pressure. Whatever you do, don't start pumping, otherwise you'll continue to produce more milk. Take an ibuprofen, if necessary, to reduce swelling, and make sure you're wearing a comfortable bra, with lots of pads and loose clothing. Change wet pads regularly and ensure you don't have anything digging into full breasts, as this can cause blocked ducts. Your milk will start to dry up and the engorgement will become less each day. Massage any lumps that appear with warm compresses to help them disperse. A supplement of lecithin can help break down blocked ducts. Speak to a herbalist or an assistant in a health-food shop for dosages.

Alternatively, you could reduce the feeds over a number of days. This is a more gentle method but it will depend on why you're stopping as to whether this is feasible. Cut one feed per day and replace it with a bottle. Your milk supply will start to reduce gradually. Use the same methods as above to relieve engorgement and, again, avoid pumping. The only problem with this last method, or potentially with either, is how your baby responds. Some babies are more difficult to wean than others. If you've been breastfeeding for a while, it might be harder to get the baby off the boob.

Because breastfeeding is more than just nutrition for a baby, they may grizzle about their perceived rejection if you attempt feeding them from a bottle. The closeness you get from breastfeeding can be quite emotional for both mother and baby, and this is where the difficulty lies. Some mothers harbour huge guilt about stopping breastfeeding, so that needs also to be addressed during the process. Try expressing a feed to begin with so that baby is still getting your breast milk. Then, while feeding from the bottle, have skin-to-skin contact and don't force the baby if they get upset.

Getting your partner to feed the baby from a bottle can separate the association to begin with. Try offering a bottle at different times of the day. Some babies may accept a bottle in the middle of the day but not in the evenings when they're tired. Offer the bottle frequently, as with weaning onto solids, it's suggested that by repeating a rejected food, the baby will eventually adapt and accept. Seek advice from an expert if you are having difficulties.

BREATHING

Just like giving birth, your body instinctively knows how to breathe. Every time you doubt your inherent amazingness and the wisdom of your physiology, take a deep breath and consider how many times a day you do that without knowing. But slow, deep breathing is your best friend when it comes to surfing the waves of **contractions** (see page 135). Just don't rock up in labour and expect to be able to breathe deeply – practise and prepare.

Take ten minutes each day to lie down, close your eyes and breathe in for a count of ten and out for ten, taking the air all the way down to your belly. Picture the air coming in through your feet and out through the top of your head.

As you do this, mentally scan your body for any knots of tension and feel them melt away. Eventually, when you're all floppy and warm, breathe normally and quietly until you feel like getting up. You may nod off – lucky you! But it's a great way to get used to the long, slow, conscious breathing that will be a handy tool in labour – and also when you're dealing with a furious two-year-old in a supermarket queue several months from now.

BREECH

In the vast majority of pregnancies, babies will be positioned with their head down, snuggly fitted into the pelvis close to birth. Their feet will be perfectly positioned to kick you in the ribs, and they'll do heavyweight-world-champion-standard jabbing into your lower uterus, occasionally making perfect contact with nerves that will send shooting pains down your legs. So, when a breech baby is identified in pregnancy or goes undiagnosed until you are in labour, your pregnancy and birth can take on a completely different hue. You might notice that I'm using my language quite carefully. There are some books that will automatically tell you that a **caesarean** birth (see page 115) is the only safe option and to consider a vaginal birth is tantamount to child abuse. That's basically bollocks. Women birthed breech babies for generations, because midwives had the skills to deliver them. Yes, some would have fared worse than if caesareans were carried out, but many more would have been born safely and without complications.

Then, as today, a vaginal birth with a breech presentation is possible in some instances. You just need to weigh up any concerns and know whom to speak to about your particular situation. It's impossible for me to tell you what would be right in your specific instance. Your medical team will need to weigh up many factors: is this your first baby? How big is it? Are you overdue? How relaxed are you about a vaginal birth? Do you intend to have more children? There are many variables that must be considered. But being informed will be vital, hence the inclusion here of wisdom from two of the country's best midwives and the very best brains when it comes to breech. Midwife, academic and researcher Shawn Walker is the UK's leading expert on breech birth, and Victoria Cochrane (MSc, BSc) is also a highly qualified specialist, as well as being a consultant midwife with a remit for normalising pregnancy and birth for all women.

This is their exclusive, expert opinion.

Shawn Walker and Victoria Cochrane on discovering your baby is breech

About a quarter of babies are breeches at 28 weeks, and most will turn. If this is your first baby, only about one-third of babies who are breech at 33 weeks will turn spontaneously; however, if you have had a head-down baby before, the chances are very good that baby will turn on his own by the start of labour. That being said, about 3–4 per cent of babies will remain breech at term.

To avoid leaving your baby's breech position undetected until you go into labour, you should pay close attention to your baby's normal pattern of movements. If you notice that he is kicking down into your vagina, or you feel a hard ball (their head) under your ribs, make sure you mention it to the midwife.

Having highlighted that skilled hands and ultrasound

scans can diagnose a breech-presenting baby in the antenatal period, it's good to keep in mind that 25 per cent are not known about until women are in labour. If this is the case, quick thinking about your choices will need to be made in a calm fashion.

Types of breech

Breech babies are fantastic dancers and get themselves into all sorts of positions, and it can be quite hard to pin them down for this reason, but there are three main types of breech presentation:

1. **Frank breech**, where your baby is folded in half like a taco, with his feet up by his face.
2. **Complete breech**, where the baby's legs are bent at the knees, and often folded over.
3. **Footling breech**, where one (or both) of the baby's legs is positioned below its bottom. This presentation usually only affects pre-term or very small breech babies, and it carries some increased risks.

Encouraging your baby to turn

From 34 weeks, the evidence indicates that using moxibustion (it looks a bit like a cigar and is filled with the Chinese herb moxa – it smells!) in combination with **acupuncture** (see page 23), and/or positional techniques such as spinning babies (see baby's position in Resources), might be successful, but you would need to talk to someone qualified to provide moxibustion and acupuncture to fully understand your options.

Should your baby be breech at 33–34 weeks and have

Breech births

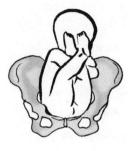 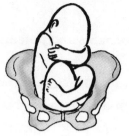 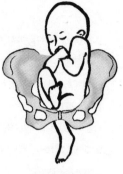

Frank breech   Complete breech   Footling breech

been in this position for some time, now is the time to start thinking and reading about the type of birth that is important to you.

External cephalic version

For all pregnant women, most maternity services will offer external cephalic version (ECV), where the baby is manually turned by a trained obstetrician or midwife, by pressing on the outside of your abdomen, from about 36–37 weeks. This is usually done with tocolysis, a medication to relax your uterus, and sometimes with spinal pain relief. In centres where vaginal breech birth is not often offered as an option, having an ECV will increase your chances of having a vaginal birth, although there is a small (1 in 200) chance of requiring an emergency c-section following the procedure. In terms of ECV, it's important to ask how frequently the individual performs this procedure, as this will affect their success rates, with most around 50 per cent when performed on a weekly basis. Should the first person not be successful, it is very reasonable for another person to try a few days to a week later.

Weighing up the benefits and potential risks

When looking at vaginal breech birth versus caesarean section, the best available evidence indicates that vaginal breech birth carries some greater risks around the time of birth for the baby compared to an elective c-section; however, the absolute risks are small. The most recent study indicated the neonatal mortality (the risk of baby dying) is about 3 in 1,000, and this included countries with maternity systems that generally do not have results as good as the UK. It is likely that the increased short-term risk of a vaginal breech birth is similar to the risks of a normal, head-down birth, but greater than c-section. The most likely adverse outcome is that baby will require resuscitation at birth and be admitted to the neonatal unit for support in the first few days of life, and this may happen for up to 1 in 20 vaginally born breech babies, versus 1 in 60 babies born by elective c-section.

On the other hand, elective c-section is associated with a greater long-term risk of non-specific medical problems in life, such as asthma, diabetes and obesity, for the child. And a scarred uterus carries greater risks in future pregnancies for both future babies and mum.

Many trusts still inform women that elective c-section is the only option for the birth of their breech baby – this is not the case!

Our advice

Take a deep breath, it's not an easy or simple decision to make, but there are pros and cons to each option: ECV, vaginal breech birth and elective c-section.

Make sure you get the support and information you deserve to make the right decision for you. You can ask to speak to the consultant midwife (ask for his or her email address/mobile number) and they should offer you an appointment to fully discuss all your options and make a plan to support you. Some trusts have developed a breech-birth service/team and your midwife can put you in touch with them. There are also online groups such as Breech Birth UK (see Resources) that provide peer support for women.

BUM

With so much going on out front when you're pregnant, it can be easy to neglect your backside for a few months and just accept the fact that you are definitely growing one baby in your belly and one in each rear cheek. But too much weight gain in pregnancy is not a good idea: big babies can be harder to squeeze out. Do yourself a favour, go easy on the three o'clock Mars Bars and get off the bus a stop sooner. (It's a rather disheartening fact that pregnant women don't need that many more calories, so check out **diet**, page 140 for some top tips.)

If you're unlucky, ignoring your bum might not be an option, due to piles. These are very common in pregnancy and are simply blood vessels in your lower rectum and anus that become inflamed and swollen. It's our pesky friend progesterone again, the hormone that relaxes body tissues. Add your newly stretchy a-hole to slackened veins and a heavy baby, and out pop some new friends. They may itch and cause pain, particularly if they make a bid for freedom and appear on the outside of your body – particularly after you've been for an uncooperative poo.

Some women even get vulva varicosities: vaginal piles (you heard it here first). You just leave these alone and avoid standing in the same position for a long period of time and do pelvic-floor exercises. These shouldn't be a barrier to a vaginal birth.

Avoiding piles

The good news is that despite it being a common occurrence during pregnancy, there are steps you can take to avoid getting piles: drink loads of water and eat fruit, veggies and seeds to keep you loose and laughing. Linseeds are particularly good and can be added to cereal or yogurt. Constipation can contribute to piles, as too much pushing and grunting increases their likelihood. Exercise to get the blood flowing and your bowels moving.

Annoyingly, on visiting the loo, it might feel as though you haven't fully emptied the tanks, and so you continue to push, putting even more pressure on the area. You may even notice some terrifying fresh blood on the tissue after you wipe. Don't panic. Be sure it's from your bottom rather than your front bottom, and then rage at Mother Nature for the gift of ensuring we truly understand the phrase 'pain in the arse'.

Some women find that holding a warm flannel against their bottom can ease the pain and discomfort. We don't suggest you do this in the office unless you have extremely understanding colleagues. You may find those wet botty wipes kinder to your tush than plain, old, unempathic toilet roll. Don't be tempted to push the piles back into the rectum while you're on the loo. If they have been hanging out for a while and are not inflamed, it might be possible to gently push them back in using a lubricating jelly or when in the bath or shower. Ask a trusted pharmacist what ointments you might be able to use in pregnancy (some creams can break down stitches and shouldn't be used). Don't be embarrassed – the chemists have heard it all before.

C is for ...

CAESAREAN SECTION

Contrary to popular belief, this procedure does not get its name because Julius Caesar was born this way. That's just one of the many fabrications that surround extracting a baby through a cut (*caesa* in Latin) in the abdomen. These also include the belief that it's the easy option, that it's risk-free, that it hurts less or that it is always a 'shame' and a sign of 'failure'. There are times when a planned caesarean is far preferable to a vaginal birth, and it is not the preserve of women 'too posh to push' (although class does complicate the issue in countries such as Brazil where it denotes wealth). Just sweep aside all you think you know about this procedure, pour yourself a cuppa and open your mind.

Firstly, language is powerful, and the language around caesareans absolutely sucks. Meeting your baby is birth, whether you do so under a Canadian waterfall or on an operating table in Birmingham. Birth is the emergence of a living being, breathing unaided by a placenta. So, let's start a revolution, drop the 'section' bit and replace it with 'birth'?

Plus, the word 'caesarean' is stupidly archaic, thought up by public schoolboys who would jest in Latin and felt all manly with a knife in their hands. If this is the alternative to a vaginal birth, then why not call it 'abdominal birth'? Personally, I like 'belly birth', but this sort of chattiness doesn't sit well in medical textbooks.

The rising rates of caesarean sections

According to the World Health Organization, no community should have an abdominal birth rate (they don't call it that – yet) of more than 10–15 per cent. In the UK, according to NHS statistics, our rate is 26 per cent: 11 per cent planned and 15 per cent emergency.

Older women are more likely to have an unplanned abdominal birth than younger women, and first-time mothers are more likely to have an unplanned abdominal birth than women having a baby for the second or subsequent time.

The reasons for this figure being so high are complex. Modern hospitals don't always facilitate the best conditions for women, who are all too often expected to birth with a **midwife** (see page 243) they do not know, rendering the whole process infinitely more difficult (but, not, of course impossible).

Also, hospitals are scared of being sued, so a culture of 'defensive practice' has emerged, meaning that it can feel safer to a maternity team to perform surgery than to give a woman the time and support that she needs to birth without it. This is actually a fallacy, unsupported by the evidence, but it is hardly surprising when wards are rushed, under-staffed and under-funded.

A lack of continuity of care means that women are passed from pillar to post without one individual taking responsibility for them. This lack of joined-up care makes the operation more likely, as such a procedure should be considered as part of a much bigger picture which the deciding doctor may not have access to.

Certain celebrities have done a good job of making a caesarean look like a doddle. Victoria Beckham demonstrating unfathomable slenderness following each of her five abdominal births helped cement the idea that it's aspirational to be 'too posh to push'.

Plus, we're getting fatter, and our babies are getting bigger. Obesity should not be an automatic signpost towards birth surgery, but all too often it is. There is a theory that our sedentary lifestyles are contributing to the fact that vaginal births are getting longer and more complicated. Our mothers kept their pelvises flexed and babies head down by scrubbing floors and squatting while doing housework. We sit in cars, at desks and recline on sofas in positions that encourage babies to slide back to back (see **occiput posterior**, page 251) or **breech** (see page 108), making a vaginal birth trickier.

The risks

Why does any of the above matter? Surely, normal birth carries risks, and so why not negate those by opting for surgery? Well, very simply, abdominal births carry more long- and short-term risks for mum and baby than a vaginal birth. This is a fact that can get shouted down in the mainstream media by women who had abdominal births and feel criticised for it. It's even forgotten by individual **obstetricians** (see page 249) viewing each birth in isolation (they may not always inform you of the risks to your longer term health, for example).

A woman who has already had an abdominal birth does not

automatically have to have another. They should be supported to have a VBAC (vaginal birth after caesarean), if that is what they want.

As always, the skill and perspective of your medical practitioner is paramount when faced with the option of an abdominal birth. According to the Royal College of Obstetricians and Gynaecologists, a fall in the number of senior obstetricians in labour wards has resulted in increased reliance on unsupervised junior doctors. Dr Maggie Blott, a consultant obstetrician at King's College Hospital, London, has been quoted as saying, 'Junior obstetricians simply do not know how to respond to complex labours except by performing caesarean sections. The result is too many caesareans are taking place, too many of which are performed by doctors who don't necessarily have enough experience to guarantee their patients' safety.'

This isn't intended to scare you. It's to equip you. Ask about the level of experience that your treating doctor has. Demand to see a consultant and get a second opinion, if time permits. Most importantly, don't opt blindly for birth in this way. As with any procedure, get your head around the short- and long-term risks before you make a decision.

Short-term risks

The need for intensive care An abdominal birth increases the chance of the mother needing to be admitted to an intensive care unit (ICU); however, this is still uncommon and happens to 9 in every 1,000 women.

Infection One in 12 women will develop an infection, despite routine use of antibiotics prior to surgery. The main sites are:

- The incision wound: signs include redness and discharge, worsening pain, a complete or partial breakdown of the scar, and a lack of healing. It's more likely to happen if you have diabetes or are overweight. Anecdotally, these are becoming more prevalent due to poor NHS postnatal care.

- The lining of your uterus (endometritis) or from any retained placental tissue. This is more likely to happen if your waters broke before labour started, or if you had lots of vaginal examinations before your caesarean. It can cause fever, womb pain, and abnormal vaginal discharge or heavy bleeding.

- Urinary tract infection. The thin tube (catheter) inserted during the operation to empty your bladder can cause infection. You might find that weeing is difficult and painful, and that it causes a burning sensation.

A blood clot This is a risk with any surgery and can be serious, depending on where the clot lodges. If it lodges in your lungs (pulmonary embolism), it can even be life threatening. Signs include a cough or shortness of breath. If you get a pain and swelling in your calf, this can be a sign of deep-vein thrombosis. Call your doctor if you notice any of these signs after your birth. Your medical team will give you preventive treatments, such as blood-thinning drugs and elastic support stockings, to improve the blood flow in your legs. You'll be encouraged to move around as soon as possible after your caesarean. This will help your circulation and reduce the risk of a clot forming.

Scar tissue A caesarean carries a risk of adhesions as you heal. These are bands of internal scar tissue that can make organs in your tummy stick to each other, or to the inside of the wall of your tummy. About half of women who have had an abdominal birth have adhesions. The scar tissue itself is not a problem, but the adhesion occurs when it sticks to other internal organs and creates complications, such as bowel blockages. These can be painful, as they limit the movement of your internal organs. They can sometimes lead to problems with bowel obstruction and fertility if they press on or block neighbouring organs.

Adhesions are common in any type of abdominal surgery, but they happen regularly with such births because of the location of the incision site. Ideally, scar tissue disappears over a period of time. But since abdominal births can decrease blood flow to certain tissues, the healing process can be interrupted, making the scarring permanent.

The more ab-births a woman has, the more likely she is to develop adhesions, which can cause problems in future pregnancies if the baby is also delivered in this way. Since the obstetrician has to cut through adhesions in addition to the rest of the skin, tissue and fat, it can take longer to get through to the baby than it took with the first birth. This can be problematic if the baby is in distress and needs to be removed immediately. Third and fourth abdominal-birth deliveries can take more than 8–18 minutes longer, respectively. Seventy-five per cent of women who have a second, experience adhesions afterwards and 83 per cent of women with four or five have them. The skill of the surgeon will have an effect, such as which layers are stitched up afterwards, and how.

Bleeding More blood is lost in a straightforward abdominal birth than in an uncomplicated vaginal birth. Most bleeding occurs during the surgery and is easily managed by the obstetrician, who may do a blood transfusion. You are more likely to lose excess blood if a prolonged period of medical induction has preceded the birth.

Injury to your bladder, bowel or ureter (the tube that connects the kidney and bladder), which may require further surgery. This is rare, and happens to about 1 woman in 1,000 in the UK.

Longer-term risks

Opening of the incision scar during a later pregnancy or labour. Once you've had an abdominal birth you're more likely to have another in future pregnancies. But this isn't always the case, and a vaginal birth after caesarean (VBAC) may be possible. The scar on the uterus can cause a weakness in the uterine wall and the stretching that occurs during pregnancy or the strong contractions of labour can cause the scar to become thin or begin to separate: scar dehiscence. But it's rare – occurring in only 0.5–2 per cent of women; however, if the uterine scar tears open, causing bleeding and other complications, it is called 'uterine rupture' and is a serious risk to both mum and baby. This happens in 1 in 300 VBAC labours, but good care and observation in labour should mean that if a rupture looks likely, a woman can have a caesarean very quickly. An experienced midwife will monitor the baby's heartbeat and mum's pulse. This, along with watching for abnormalities, such as bleeding or pain that lasts between contractions, allows an early warning of potentially serious problems.

Problems with the placenta The surgery increases your risk of having problems with the placenta in subsequent pregnancies, including: placenta praevia, (the growth of the placenta low in the uterus, blocking the cervix); placenta accreta (the placenta attaches itself too deeply and too firmly into the uterus); placenta increta (the placenta attaches itself even more deeply into the muscle wall of uterus); and placenta percreta (the placenta attaches itself and grows through the uterus, sometimes extending to nearby organs, such as the bladder). In these conditions, the placenta doesn't completely separate from the uterus after you give birth. This can cause dangerous bleeding. These conditions happen in about 1 in 530 births each year and may sometimes require a hysterectomy.

Postnatal depression Medical studies have indicated that postnatal depression is more common after abdominal births than for women who deliver vaginally. We don't really know why, but women often report that they didn't feel involved with the birth or that there is a sense that they failed, as they weren't able to birth vaginally. Remember, they are life-saving and – most of the time – are completely necessary; however, don't underestimate the effects of your hormones on your emotional well-being. In the case of an abdominal birth, these hormones are not generated in the same quantities as they are during and after a vaginal birth. Most significant is **oxytocin** (see page 257), which helps with the release of the placenta and afterbirth. It also initiates lactation and helps kick-start the bonding process between mother and baby. It also helps the mother forget the painful process she just went through. An abdominal-birth mum doesn't benefit from the presence of these hormones in the same quantities, so be mindful of this and don't beat yourself up if you're feeling down.

Skin-to-skin contact as soon as possible after birth can help to kick-start your happy hormones. If the baby has emerged screaming and in good health, there is no reason why he shouldn't be able to be put straight onto your chest.

Scheduling your birth at no earlier than 39 weeks seems to help limit the chances of depression. Many doctors don't want women to go into labour before surgery, especially if you've had a previous abdominal birth. But if this is your first and your doctor does not express concern, booking your surgery as close to your expected delivery date is important; not only for you but also for your baby. If possible, waiting until you go into labour is also to be considered. This way, you know that your baby is ready to be born and you may wish to experience early labour. Ask your doctors (using BRAINS – see page 279) for the pros and cons of doing this in your individual circumstances.

What about future pregnancies? Some studies have suggested that abdominal births can cause secondary infertility but the research is unclear and needs more investigation; however, it does appear that women who have one c-section have fewer subsequent children. This is just something to consider if a larger family is important to you.

Risks to your baby

- About one in 50 babies is accidentally nicked with the doctor's scalpel, but this usually heals without causing any harm.
- Breathing difficulties – the most common problem affecting babies born via the belly is difficulty breathing, although this is mainly an issue for babies born prematurely. For babies born at or after 39 weeks, this breathing risk is reduced significantly to a level similar to that associated with vaginal delivery. Straight after the birth, and in the first few days of life, your baby may breathe abnormally fast. This is called transient tachypnoea. Most

newborns with transient tachypnoea recover completely within two or three days. Skin-to-skin contact can help to regulate your baby's temperature and breathing. If you think your baby is experiencing breathing difficulties, call 999 straightaway.

Medical reasons for having a pre-labour, planned abdominal birth

- Position of the baby – abnormal positioning inside the womb, such as the **breech** position (see page 108), can make it more difficult to fit through the birth canal. But breech does not automatically indicate the need for surgery.
- Multiple births – twins (or more). One or more of the babies may be in an abnormal breech position (bottom or feet first), or two or more of the babies might share a placenta, which means a caesarean section, as it increases the risk of complications in labour; however, good, continuous care might mean that a vaginal birth is possible with twins, depending on any other risk factors antenatally or during labour.
- Pelvis size and shape – most women have the same inlet and outlet, but the shape of the pelvis can cause problems. If you had an abdominal birth first-time round based on assumptions about pelvis shape and size, you can have an MRI scan to establish if this is the case. Obviously this is expensive, so you won't be routinely offered it. I highly recommend all women have a pelvic-alignment assessment with a skilled physiotherapist. This can be extremely valuable, especially if you have ever had a pelvic injury.
- Working out the exact relationship between pelvis and

babies is a very inexact science. Some women of small stature birth huge 4.5kg babies easily, and others struggle to release a small baby. This can be because of the drugs that are on board or the position of the mother. Simply being told your baby is 'too big for you' must always be questioned and is worth seeking a second opinion.

- Placenta praevia – when the placenta blocks the exit of the womb.
- Infection – if you have certain viral infections, such as a first attack of genital herpes, you may not want to risk transferring the virus to your baby.
- A medical condition – for example, a heart problem – might put you at risk during a normal delivery, or other organ problems that mean it's in your best interests to stop being pregnant.
- Restricted growth of the baby – some babies who are not growing well in the womb have a higher risk of dying or being ill around the time of birth, so a swift and calm release of the baby through the abdomen is a good idea.

What happens in an abdominal birth?

For a pre-labour, planned or elective operation, you will go into hospital the night before or, more commonly, very early on the morning of the operation. Take your **birth bag** (see page 65) and be excited! You'll have routine blood tests and take a medicine to reduce the acidity in your stomach.

The final preparations will involve changing into a hospital gown, having a bikini shave along the top line, if necessary (or you can do this at home before you leave), and removing nail varnish, glasses or contact lenses, and jewellery.

You'll have a catheter inserted into your urethra, which is uncomfortable but shouldn't be especially painful. The material is very soft and the width of a phone-charging wire. This keeps the bladder empty, which minimises the risk of it being nicked by the scalpel.

You will have a name band on your wrist. You may also need to take some clothes for your baby with you to theatre.

You will then be taken to the operating theatre. If you are having a spinal or **epidural** anaesthetic (see page 155), your birth partner will be able to stay with you during the birth, but will have to change into theatre clothes including a fetching hat. If you are going to have a general anaesthetic (this happens in 10 per cent of cases for specific, rare medical reasons), your birth partner will usually be asked to stay outside the room.

Don't be freaked out by the number of people in the room – this can be as many as 12, including midwives, paediatricians and anaesthetists. You will lie on an operating table with a low curtain across your chest so that you can't see what the doctor is doing. You can ask to have this removed.

The procedure

The surgeon makes a horizontal cut across the belly just above the pubic area. Your muscles aren't cut – they are moved to the side. The womb (uterus) and amniotic sac are opened and the baby is delivered. You will probably feel some tugging – but no pain. If you feel any pain, make sure you shout about it! It may be that in this, extremely rare, circumstance, you will be given an instant general anaesthetic. Fluid from the baby's mouth and nose are removed by suction. The umbilical cord is cut (you can request delayed **cord clamping** – see page 137). The team will make sure that the infant's breathing is normal and other vital signs are stable.

Removing the baby can be as quick as 5–15 minutes, but the stitching can take up to an hour. This will usually be one continuous stitch with beads at either end, or special skin staples that will need to be removed later.

If your baby is known to be well (if, for example, the abdominal birth is due to your health condition), there is no reason why you can't have your child straight on your chest and onto the breast. This is a special moment. There is no need to have your baby weighed straight away or whisked off to have a nappy put on. Make sure your team knows if you want instant skin-to-skin. You can still do a **birth plan** (see page 71) for an abdominal birth, and this could be included.

After the surgery

Afterwards, you will be moved out of the operating theatre to another room called a 'recovery room', but exact procedures differ between hospitals. There, a midwife will monitor you to make sure that there are no problems until you have recovered sufficiently to be taken to the postnatal ward. If you wish to breastfeed, the midwife should help you get your baby latched on. This will help get your happy hormones flowing and help seed the baby's **microbiome** (see page 243). You might feel cold, shaky and nauseous. These are mainly the side effects of the drugs and will wear off. They may also be due to your profound relief of being out of theatre and in bed with your precious little angel! If you weren't able to have skin-to-skin contact in the theatre, do so now and enjoy every second.

You will be given a painkiller that lasts for several hours. It is also a good idea to wear tight stockings and/or be given medication to reduce the risk of getting blood clots (thrombosis).

You will stay in the hospital for two or three nights and then be sent home with painkillers. Don't be a martyr – take them! It will hurt to cough or sneeze; holding a pillow against your abdomen may help. Compression garments may also be comforting on your belly. The pain will be worse for the first week but should soon improve.

You may feel like lying still, but getting up off the bed and walking around as soon as the doctor or midwife tells you to is a good idea. This is one of the few times when I'd say, 'Don't argue, and do as you're told!' It will get the blood pumping, thereby reducing the risk of clots, and blood flow to the abdomen aids repair.

Healing

You won't have as much postpartum bleeding as with a vaginal delivery (since the vaginal cavity is wiped clean at the time of your surgery), but bleeding will still happen. After all, your uterine wall has to heal itself after the placenta has been detached, and your blood vessels are responding to the dip in hormone levels. Plus, that thick lining that grew to support the baby throughout your pregnancy will need to shed itself in the weeks after your delivery. Don't worry though – any bleeding should be light and only last about six weeks, max.

Be prepared that your scar might freak you out for a while. It's unusual to find your body changed in this way, but, over time, it will flatten and fade, remaining as a mummy battle scar to prove you did something amazing. After it has been allowed to air as much as possible over the first six weeks, you can use scar-fading ointments or oils such as Weleda (see Resources).

Don't be surprised if you get bizarre wind pains in your shoulders after delivery. When your bowels become sluggish after surgery, the resulting gas can press on the diaphragm, and that pain can extend to the shoulders. Your midwife might offer you some drugs to ease the wind. Or you can try walking around as soon as possible. Weirdly, this may not be the only cause of postsurgical shoulder pain. It is the result of referred pain: pain that's actually being caused in another part of the body (in this case, your uterus), but felt somewhere else, because of the way your nerves react. Abdominal births teach you all sorts of things about the human body.

Like any mum who has had a vaginal birth, you will find going for your first poo a tad terrifying. Just try to relax: you will not burst your stitches. But drink water and consider taking a poo softener, as the drugs can render your bowels a little uncooperative.

Emergency abdominal birth

This follows the exact same chronology as a planned operation, but there will be a sense of urgency for everyone involved. It will be difficult, but try to breathe slowly and deeply to keep your heart rate steady and to get plenty of oxygen to your baby. **Hypnobirthing** (page 206) comes into its own in this scenario.

You still have options

Too few women know that they have choices, even with a medicalised birth. In response to women reporting feeling unhappy after a surgical birth, more and more obstetricians are now offering what is called either a 'gentle', 'slow', 'natural' or 'woman-centred' caesarean.

These small changes might seem irrelevant, or even silly, as you see them here on the page, but women who are respected, treated with kindness and have the significance of their birth day recognised have happier births.

You will have to ask around for an obstetrician who supports your wishes. This is not yet standard practice because of the way that obstetricians are trained. Don't be fobbed off. Your day is important. And with every woman who asks, the wheel towards putting women at the heart of their care slowly turns.

The gentle/natural caesarean

In this kind of procedure, one or more of the following choices are observed:

- The room is kept calm and quiet. There is no chit-chat over the woman's head about the football scores. The atmosphere is respectful.
- Music of the parents' choice can be played (this should be standard in all abdominal births).
- The screen is lowered during the birth or immediately afterwards, so that mum and partner can watch the baby being born.
- The baby is born more slowly, mimicking the way fluid is squeezed from the lungs in the process of a vaginal birth.
- The parents can discover the sex of the baby themselves rather than it being announced.
- There is a delay in cord clamping.
- The ECG dots are attached to mum's back instead of her chest so that she can have skin-to-skin contact immediately with baby.
- The IV (intravenous) line is placed in mum's non-dominant hand so that it is easier for her to touch and caress her baby.

Florence's story

I had read almost every book ever written about pregnancy while gestating my daughter, but I neglected to read anything about caesareans. My daughter had to be delivered a few weeks early due to my own pre-existing health complication, but she was absolutely fine in utero, cooking gently. Having been wisely advised to question medical opinion about these things, I was assured the caesarean would save both our lives, and so it happened pretty much right away. I was furious with the timings ('I haven't put the sheets on the cot!'), but from start to finish, the entire process was incredibly, charmingly, surprisingly – civilised.

I would imagine an emergency caesarean might be very different, and I salute the bravery and stoicism of women in that difficult situation. But it doesn't always have to be difficult or painful or frightening or 'non-bonding'. Of course, I was nervous, I was excited and full of anticipation and fear of the unknown. But the overarching impression of the day was of jovial calm.

The much-dreaded spinal block was administered with confidence and sensitivity; the birth itself was quick and not painful (it was weird and uncomfortable and nauseating but I figured that was only to be expected); I was able to have skin-to-skin straightaway and put my baby to the breast almost immediately; my husband was by my side for every second of every minute and was able to do a cord cutting, plus skin-to-skin under his (frankly quite attractive) blue scrubs.

The physical recovery was much easier than had been suggested. I was a little sore in a muscular way and a little itchy around my stitches (well, they had to, ahem, shave a little bit down there), but it was all very manageable and I was up and wandering about that same afternoon. For us it was the perfect way to welcome our baby into the world and I'm overwhelmingly grateful to everyone who made it her birthday.

CALMNESS

If there is one state of mind that will help you towards a happy birth, this is it. Keeping your pulse steady and your happy hormones flowing will provide the optimal physiological conditions for labour. However things roll, you will cope better if you're able to remain chilled. **Oxytocin** (see page 257) explains why this state of mind is so important, especially if you don't intend to birth at home. Here are my top tips for staying calm.

- Practise **Hypnobirthing** (see page 206) in the weeks and months before birth.
- On arrival at your birthplace, let your partner do most of the talking.
- Keep your headphones on and listen to a downloaded relaxation track.
- Keep your eyes closed as much as possible (without walking into doors).
- Breathe slowly and deeply – exhaling longer than inhaling.
- Internally track the sensations in your muscles from your toes to the top of your head – when you find tension, release it through long breaths.
- Have a trusted birth attendant that you know.

- Lower the lights.
- Request that interruptions are kept to a minimum.
- Don't concern yourself with what is going on in the room around you. Zone out if your partner and midwife are chatting about the weather.
- Have a few positive phrases that you can tell yourself over and over. Reassure yourself that you're in a developed world with great medical support.
- Try a birth pool (see **water birth**, page 317), even if only for several minutes. Water is inherently calming.
- Remember that every contraction is a step closer to your baby.

CAUL

Some babies are born in the membrane sac or caul as it's, er, called. Traditionally, before medics got busy with hooks to break membrane sacks, many more babies would have been born this way. Nevertheless, the relative rarity of such births bestowed such babies and their cauls with superstitious powers of good fortune. In Charles Dickens's *David Copperfield*, the eponymous hero's own caul is auctioned off as a talisman to protect against drowning. Copperfield describes how he felt at being present at the auction of his own caul:

I remember to have felt quite uncomfortable and confused, at part of myself being disposed of in that way. The caul was won, I recollect, by an old lady with a hand-basket ... It is a fact which will be long remembered as remarkable down there, that she was never drowned, but died, triumphantly in bed, at ninety-two.

Even as late as the 1950s, people still believed in the powers of such cauls. In 1954 in Banbury a midwife offered a new mother the high price of £10 for her child's caul, as she wanted it for a sailor; however, if your baby is born in this way in the twenty-first century, your midwife may look askance if you ask to take the caul home as a protective amulet for your booze-cruise ferry crossings

CERVIX

Your cervix sits at the bottom of your uterus and stops your baby falling out. It plays a huge role in **labour** (see page 232). During pregnancy, it is long, hard and closed tight shut. But as labour approaches, it softens, shortens and eventually opens and disappears – this is called effacement and dilation. In the language of birth, you are likely to feel an instinctive pushing sensation when your cervix is 10cm dilated. After this, your baby transitions down, into the birth canal and eventually out of your vagina and into the real world. Of course, it would be ridiculous to take this 10cm measurement literally. It's a rough estimation of an average cervix, which enables practitioners to guesstimate the duration of a labour. During a vaginal examination, midwives assess how much cervix remains – this is as informative to them as how wide the dilatation is. The cervix should be fully closed again at your six-week check. Your cervix has a good memory and will probably efface and dilate more quickly with each pregnancy and birth.

CHAMPAGNE

There are few situations that are not improved by a glass of bubbles. Stick a tiny bottle of champers in the hospital bag – it's a visual reminder that you're not on your way to war – you're heading towards the celebration of a new life! Toast each other and the innate wonderfulness after giving birth. I could tell you about women so stressed in early labour that they were prescribed a couple of sips to calm them down. But that would be inappropriate, so I'd never do that.

CONTRACTIONS

Even if you know nothing about birth, the chances are you've heard about contractions. These are simply the tightening and releasing of your uterine muscles to release your baby downwards. They are nothing to be feared.

Some women find early contractions (Hypnobirthers call them 'surges') intense and tiring; they struggle to eat or get any rest. Others find them manageable and are able to bounce on a Swiss ball, keep busy or calm enough to ignore them. Try to stay positive. This early stage can be a bit demoralising if it lasts for more than a day or two, and can make real labour feel like you still have a mountain to climb. But eat, drink and rest when you can. Make sure everyone around you is filling you with positive messages of encouragement. Between contractions you will feel either completely normal and totally pain-free or excited, happy and a little high on your own hormonal cocktail. Remember to observe your body and how it feels – it's pretty special. Try to be mindful of those lovely in-between moments rather than clinging to the side of the chair and dreading the next sensation.

You may be the type of person who would like to time their contractions over the course of 30 minutes. You may feel reassured by keeping track of your progress. There are apps for this, and men seem particularly happy to have this important job. Note the time at the start of a contraction then at the end of the contraction, and then the time at the start of the next contraction, and so on; for example, in early labour, you might have a contraction every 7 minutes, lasting 40 seconds, giving you a rest between contractions of 6 minutes and 20 seconds.

Your midwife might ask how frequent they are, so timing them can be useful. Your **birth centre** (see page 68) or hospital will give you rough guidelines about when to come in. The midwife on the end of the phone will want to talk to you rather than your partner, as she can tell a lot from the sound of your voice.

When to depart for the hospital

Early on, you'll probably be able to talk through your contractions, and continue with your normal routine. If there is one major tip I can offer regarding labour, it is to stay at home for as long as you possibly can. Do not rush to your place of birth unless you have been medically advised to do so.

Whatever you want to happen in labour, it is more likely to be smoother, with fewer interventions if you stay at home until labour is properly established with strong, regular contractions. If you want an epidural, they are more likely to give you one soon if you arrive in established labour. Starting labour by yo-yoing back and forth to hospital can be tiring and demoralising as explained in **Hypnobirthing** (see page 206).

Once labour is established (you are 3–4cm dilated), contractions may come every 3–4 minutes, and last between 60 and 90 seconds. But between them you will feel completely normal, even, perhaps, a little high on endorphins. You will be able to talk, move around, have a drink and prepare yourself for the next contraction.

CORD CLAMPING

The umbilical cord is a sinewy, veiny, tough little snake that provides all nutrients and oxygen to your baby through their belly button. When the baby is born, the cord is cut, leaving about a 2.5cm stump, which is then clamped with a white plastic peg (a bit like those ones that are used to keep cereal fresh).

Each placenta has one vein (taking nutrition to the baby) and two arteries (which take away waste products) attached to the baby. They are surrounded by a thick watery jelly that prevents them being compressed. In about 1.5 per cent of all pregnancies, there will be only one artery, which can cause a slight increase in growing smaller babies or stillbirth. In this instance you'll be monitored carefully.

For the last 50–60 years, cutting the cord has been a really big deal: it can be seen as a masculine thing to do, a symbolic act with shiny scissors. Don't think too much about it, as you may get quite cross: severing the cord too soon after birth is now viewed as bad practice which has not benefitted babies.

Once your baby is born, the placenta and cord continue their function in transferring cord blood to your baby. He is using his lungs for the very first time and yet the cord is commonly cut before the baby has taken its first breath. This can deprive your baby of at least 30 per cent of their intended blood volume, and babies can gain more than 200g in their first five minutes if the cord is left unclamped. The cord blood contains a high concentration of stem cells, which are valuable for human beings throughout their lives. Babies who have immediate cord clamping have a greater incidence of iron deficiency anaemia due to red cells being left behind.

NICE guidance published at the end of 2014 recommends

delaying cord clamping for at least one minute unless the baby's heart rate is less than 60bpm and remaining slow.

Write your request on your **birth plan** (see page 71) and ask your midwife if delayed cord clamping is routine in your birth setting.

D is for . . .

DIAMORPHINE/PETHIDINE

These pain-relieving drugs were very fashionable in the 1960s and 1970s, but got a bad press for the fact that women were basically giving birth smacked off their tits on opium and it was affecting the baby's breathing directly after birth. The increased popularity of epidurals in the 1980s and 1990s rendered the use of pethidine quite rare, but recently there has been an increase in its use. If given at the right time in the right dose, diamorphine/pethidine can be a brilliant way of allowing a labouring woman some much-needed rest and thereby avoiding or delaying the need for an epidural. On the other hand, a more sceptical view might explain its re-emergence as a consequence of under-staffed maternity wards: women on diamorphine are sleepy and don't require as much one-to-one midwifery attention. It's a great way of shutting women up.

Nevertheless, there are many instances of women who credit diamorphine with allowing them a great birth. It is given by injection into your thigh by a midwife (in 50mg or 100mg doses, with repeat doses after between one hour and three hours if it isn't having an effect). As it can make you feel nauseous, it will often be combined with an anti-sickness drug.

If you would like to have diamorphine on hand at a **home birth** (see page 197), you will need to have it prescribed by the GP, and you will be responsible for collecting, storing and disposing of it safely. But speak to your midwives, as some will not be comfortable using it due to the risk of it affecting baby's breathing immediately after birth.

As with any drug, it has potential risks and side effects. Here is everything you need to know:

When is the best time to have diamorphine?

Have it too early and you are more likely to graduate to an epidural when it wears off and the sensations become too intense too quickly. If you have it too close to birth, it can affect your baby. It is best used if you have had a long, early labour and would benefit from some rest or sleep. It can be useful during the latter part of dilating but before you start to push. Unlike an epidural, it doesn't seem to slow the birth down if you're already in established labour with contractions coming thick and fast.

NHS protocol says that you cannot use a birth pool or bath during labour within two hours of a dose of diamorphine.

What are the disadvantages of diamorphine?

- It won't entirely block labour pain and may make you feel spaced out and less in control of your labour.
- One in three women finds such opiate drugs unpleasant and – ironically – make it more difficult to cope with the sensations of labour.

- Rarely, it may make you feel so drowsy that your breathing slows and you need oxygen through a face mask.
- It can make you feel sick or vomit, even if you have an anti-sickness drug.
- It may make you feel dizzy, elated or depressed.
- It crosses the placenta and may affect your baby's breathing or make them drowsy for several days, particularly if your labour develops more quickly than anticipated and your baby is born within two hours of you having the drug.
- Breastfeeding can be affected, as diamorphine might affect your baby's ability to rout and suck for a few days.

▪ DIET

Don't think about weight loss at a time like this. Your diet is suddenly important due to the fact that that what goes in your mouth is shared between you and your gorgeous little baby. Neglecting this fact (within reason: I'm sure babies enjoy the odd bag of Quavers) is not cool or clever. Just making one or two healthier choices a day will make a huge difference to your well-being during and after your pregnancy.

Jessica Scott (BA Hons DipCnm) first came to me as a pregnant mum-to-be, but is now on her way to baby number two and hosts both our pregnancy nutrition sessions and our postnatal weaning course. She is a fully qualified nutritionist at the top of her game, and I adore everything she says. Here is her advice.

Jessica Scott on pregnancy nutrition

Looking after yourself during preconception, pregnancy and breastfeeding is invaluable. A healthy diet and lifestyle can not only help prevent potential problems experienced during pregnancy, but it can also give your baby the best chance of being healthy, both at birth and long into the future. Medical research has proved beyond doubt that a healthy diet and lifestyle make conception easier and reduce miscarriage risk. Plus, the environment of your womb has an enormous effect on the future health and intellectual development of your baby.

It is also important for you. Nature ensures that your baby will always take priority over your needs when it comes to taking goodness from your food. If you are low in crucial vitamins or minerals, it will be you that suffers the most, and it is important to stay strong and healthy during pregnancy.

This does not mean, however, that the 'eating for two' myth is true. In fact, you only need an extra 100–300kcal per day (300kcal being in the last trimester). This should mainly come from extra protein and not from that extra helping of pasta or the mid-afternoon carrot cake!

General eating tips

- Try to eat a rainbow of colour every day. Each vibrant colour of fruit and vegetables contains a different set of nutrients; therefore, by eating a variety you can be sure to be covering most of your nutritional needs.
- Avoid white carbohydrates and sugary foods. Sometimes when tired these can feel like the

easiest way to a pick-me-up, but in fact they spike your blood sugar, which is followed by an almighty slump that will leave you feeling much more tired. It also increases the risk of gestational diabetes.

- Focus your diet on complex carbohydrates, vegetables, fruit and proteins.
- Eating little and often is sensible, as it keeps blood sugars balanced, energy levels high and helps with morning sickness.
- Make sure you are eating lots of nourishing foods. Cold raw food in winter is not very nurturing to a growing baby. Soups, stews and root vegetable mash are great. Be kind to your body: warm and nourishing is key.
- Eat seasonal foods; they not only have higher nutrients, but they are also cheaper and so much tastier.

Foods to avoid
- Caffeine – no more than 200mg per day, which is the equivalent of two mugs of instant coffee or half a large espresso-based coffee, such as a latte, bought from a coffee chain.
- Alcohol.
- The following *should be avoided* due to the risk of salmonella, listeria or toxoplasmosis, which are all food-borne illnesses that could have a dangerous effect on your unborn baby:

  1. Soft cheeses with white rind (unless cooked)
  2. Blue cheese (unless cooked)

3. Pâté
4. Raw or partially cooked eggs
5. Liver
6. Cured meat and salami (unless cooked)
7. Raw or undercooked meat

- The following should be avoided because of the high
  levels of mercury, dioxins and PCBs (pollutants) that
  occur in these fish:

1. Marlin, shark or swordfish
2. Fresh tuna, salmon or other oily fish (limit to two
    portions per week max.) because of the potential
    PCB contamination. Sardines and anchovies
    are packed with vitamins and are least affected
    by pollution, but the pre-packed varieties can
    contain a lot of salt.

On the following pages you'll find a guide to why you need to eat
certain food sources and the nutrients they provide.

Note: The chart does not include calcium because although it is
also very important in pregnancy, our bodies naturally increase
absorption by 45 per cent during pregnancy, so as long as you are
eating a balanced diet, your needs should be met.

INCREASED NUTRITIONAL NEEDS

Protein	
Why?	The most important element for building and growing new life
	Needs increase by 6–10g per day (1 boiled egg = about 6g)
	Protein is also great because it keeps blood sugars balanced and keeps energy levels up
Food sources	Beans, chicken, eggs, fish, game, pulses (peas, beans and lentils), quinoa, red meat
Essential fats	
Why?	Omega fats, but omega-3s especially, as they play an essential role in the development of a baby's brain, retina and nervous system
Food sources	Omega-3s in anchovies, flaxseeds, fresh tuna, halibut, mackerel, salmon, sardines and walnuts
	Omega-6s in almonds, Brazil nuts, cashew nuts, chia seeds, pecan nuts, pistachio nuts, poultry, pumpkin seeds, rapeseed oil, sesame seeds, sunflower oil, sunflower seeds, vegetable oil

Food sources	Omega-9s in avocado, almonds, cashew nuts, cold-pressed olive oil, hazelnuts, sesame oil
Folic acid	
Why?	For DNA synthesis and cell replication Prevents neural tube defects It is very important in the first few weeks of pregnancy
Food sources	Asparagus, beans, broccoli, spinach
Iron	
Why?	Extra iron is needed to expand maternal red cell production It supplies foetal and placenta tissues However, beware of taking extra iron supplements unnecessarily, as too much iron is not good for us. Usually the excess is excreted through our period, but this is not possible during pregnancy If prescribed iron, increase its absorption by taking with vitamin C; limit tea and coffee, which block its absorption and take away from meal times
Food sources	Beef, lentils, kale, kidney beans, olives, sesame seeds, soya beans, spinach

Zinc	
Why?	Key for the growing foetus and development learning Low levels are linked to spinal bifida and low birth weight
Food sources	Beef, cashew nuts, lentils, oysters, pumpkin seeds, quinoa, sardines, sesame seeds
Magnesium	
Why?	Needed to form bone, protein and fatty acids A muscle relaxant It is great if you are suffering from tension or stress It can prevent muscle cramps and restless leg It helps with sleep problems And it works a dream for constipation!
Food sources	Black beans, cashew nuts, pumpkin seeds, quinoa, rocket, sesame seeds, sunflower seeds, spinach, watercress

Iodine	
Why?	Crucial for thyroid function Low thyroid function can have serious impact on infant development The larger your boobs, the greater your need!
Food sources	Cod, scallops, salmon, sardines (2 portions maximum per week), sea vegetables, yogurt

Beta-carotene (for vitamin A)	
Why?	Vitamin A is crucial for reproduction, differentiation of cells and eyes However, too much vitamin A can be toxic and cause birth defects, so avoid processed foods with 'added' vitamin A Beta-carotene converts to vitamin A when needed, so by increasing beta-carotene-rich foods you will get enough vitamin A without any risk
Food sources	Anything yellow and orange Apricot, butternut squash, carrot, mango, melon, sweet potato, yellow pepper

B vitamins Especially B_1, B_2, B_6, B_{12}	
Why?	These are easily depleted when you are stressed and are often depleted in pregnancy Crucial for energy and can help with mood swings
Food sources	Avocado, brown rice, kale, marmite, white fish, yogurt

Supplements

Please be aware that you get what you pay for with supplements, so I would always recommend a good-quality brand preferably from either an independent health shop, or a reliable online supplier. On the whole a good, varied diet is preferable to taking supplements, but you might feel reassured by taking a good-quality, pre-natal multivitamin.

Omega-3 is best absorbed through two portions of oily fish per week, but if you don't like fish, these brain-building nutrients must be taken in a pregnancy-friendly brand:

- **A good-quality pre-natal multivitamin** will ensure most of your needs above are met.
- **An Omega-3** supplement with good levels of DHA. Although oily fish is a good source of Omega-3, due to so much mercury and pollutants

it is best avoided in high quantities in pregnancy, so it is recommended to supplement.

- **Iron** Although you don't want to over-supplement with iron unless prescribed, it is important to keep levels up, especially for the birth, as it will help with recovery time. If deficient, Solgar Gentle Iron, Floradex and Spatone sachets (available at all pharmacists) are less constipating than some supplements that doctors prescribe.
- **Magnesium** Take magnesium citrate. To resolve constipation or improve sleep, take 400mg per day (if you're using it to improve sleep, take it in the evening). For cramp or restless leg, take 400mg per day. To maintain levels, take 200mg per day.

Other good pregnancy tips

- Dandelion tea is great for low blood pressure (**note:** do not take if your blood pressure is high).
- Raspberry leaf tea tones and strengthens the uterus in preparation for birth; drink it in the final trimester.
- Flaxseeds are great for keeping your bowels moving.
- Kefir is a fermented yogurt drink that contains billions of probiotics; it is great not only for the immune system, which can be depleted in pregnancy, but also for making sure your gut is full of healthy bacteria (see **microbiome**, page 243). This will not only be beneficial to your baby during pregnancy but also for the birth and breastfeeding. It can be purchased online or in health-food stores.

Cow kefir tends to me more palatable, but goat kefir is great too, especially for anyone with a cow's milk intolerance. Drink 150–200ml per day.

◼ DOULA

You may not have heard of such a thing, but doulas can be every pregnant woman's best friend. Unlike an **independent midwife** (see page 243), doulas are not clinically trained as such, but offer the all-important role of giving you a trusted companion before, during and after birth to keep you calm and get that **oxytocin** (see page 257) flowing. Doulas feel drawn to supporting mothers and families because they think women are wonderful. A good doula will make you feel great about yourself, which can be a part of creating warm, proud memories of pregnancy, birth and early parenthood.

But don't take my word for it; listen to doula Olivia Southey, who shares her wisdom about when and why you might consider using a doula in pregnancy and beyond.

Olivia Southey on doulas

What does a doula do? It can be hard to list exactly what a doula does, because all doulas are a little bit different. Some are cuddly, some are kick-ass, some cook a mean casserole, some will pop the cork on your champagne. Some are mums who have recently had babies, some are grandmothers, some have not had children but might do great work with pregnant women as yoga teachers or acupuncturists. The important thing here is that there will be a doula out there who is a great match for you and who makes you feel safe, happy and listened to. You should be able to ask anything or do anything with your doula and really be yourself, knowing that she has your back. This is important, because it is so helpful to feel uninhibited while you are giving birth.

Where good doulas are similar is that they are all passionate about helping mothers to have positive, lovingly supported experiences of birth. They take the time to build trust and find out what you want and need for the birth of your child. They may be fond of babies, but they put you first. A doula will not give you medical advice or influence what you choose to do, but she can give you good balanced information and practical support to help you be more comfortable during labour.

As well as birth doulas there are postnatal doulas who come and work with you once your baby is born, supporting your adjustment to motherhood, letting you rest, listening to you, helping with light housework and generally empowering you to be the mum you want to be.

How can a doula help you?
The presence of a doula has been shown by research to make a real difference to your birth experience. It is called 'the doula effect'. Women who are supported by doulas have:

- Lower rates of caesarean births
- Lower rates of instrumental births
- Lower rates of induced labour
- Shorter labours (not necessarily short)
- A more positive reported experience of birth
- Increased breastfeeding rates

If you are feeling anxious about the birth, or you have had a difficult previous birth, a doula can help to prepare you so that you feel confident in your choices and your ability to cope positively, no matter how your labour unfolds. And the less fear and tension you are feeling, the easier you are making birth for yourself.

Doulas are different from other birth partners because they are not normally part of your close family or social circle. They are a bit more neutral than that and will unswervingly support your choices. Birth is an intimate time, but a doula does not interfere with the role that your partner will play during birth if you are planning for them to be with you. In fact a doula is a brilliant support for partners, as she has good birth knowledge and creates a peaceful, reassuring atmosphere.

Birth can be emotional and tiring for partners, and knowing that they can have a quick cup of tea (or a wee) without leaving you alone, and that the doula will suggest ways to genuinely help you, will enable your nearest and dearest to relax and focus on you better. And the more relaxed your partner is the more relaxed you will be too – stress is contagious.

Ideally, your doula will also create a good relationship with the midwives who are looking after you during birth. This adds to the positivity around you, protecting that magical **oxytocin** (see page 257).

Another time that doulas can be particularly beneficial is if you don't have your own family close by to support you, or if you are a solo parent. Having someone who is dedicated to you and your best interests can smooth the journey to motherhood and help you take time for the joyful bits and get support with any challenges.

Find out more

If you think that a birth doula might be a good idea, what do you do next?

Meet a few doulas who work in your area and get your partner to meet them too. You can find doulas via the Internet (see Resources) or through pregnancy groups, antenatal classes, a recommendation or a Google search. All doulas will come for a free, no-pressure conversation before you decide whether or not you are going to hire them.

Once you find a doula you click with, she will normally give you a contract or letter of agreement for your work together. Doulas normally take a deposit when you book them, and collect the rest of their fee either when they go on call for you or after the birth. Clarity is the key to a great experience, so before you commit to working together, make sure you talk about what you can expect from her in terms of number of visits before and after the birth, length of time she will be on call, whether she will come to appointments with you and anything else you would like to know.

After you have decided to work together, your doula will come to visit you several times before your birth. You might discuss your birth plan, your hopes and concerns around pregnancy and birth, any previous pregnancies or births, practical plans and how you would like any other birth partners to support you.

When you are 37 or 38 weeks pregnant, your doula will go on call for you. That means that no matter what time of day or night you go into labour, you can call her, and when you want her support, she will come. She will stay with you (unless you agree that she will come back when labour is more established) until your baby has been born and you are all settled and comfortable.

After the birth your doula will remain in touch with you to make sure you are coping well in the early days. She will come to visit you either once or several times, depending on her way of working, to continue that trusted support. She will talk through your birth with you, listening to how you feel about it, to bring the birth chapter to a close.

Then you may be happy to continue without a doula, or you can find a postnatal doula to support you during early motherhood.

Costs

Doulas charge variable fees depending on location, experience and the package on offer. Doulas who are working within Doula UK are either 'mentored' or 'recognised'.

A mentored doula has completed an approved preparation course and may have other relevant experience. While working for her first four to six clients she has access to the support and guidance of an experienced doula. Her clients will submit confidential feedback to her mentor after working with her. She will normally charge in the range of £200–£450 per birth.

Once a doula has gone through the mentoring process and is more experienced, she will charge anything between £600 and £2,000. Prices tend to reflect geographical area and level of experience.

Some doulas charge separately for travel, some include all their expenses in their fee.

Doula UK runs an access fund for vulnerable mothers who cannot afford the doula support they need.

E is for ...

▓ EPIDURAL

There are two ways to completely stop labour pains: ·

1. Getting the baby out
2. An epidural

It's worth considering that epidurals can slow labour down – hence extending the length of time it takes to get the baby out. But some women find giving birth so painful, or are in such need of some relief after a long, early labour that an epidural becomes their best option. There is nobody waiting in hospital receptions to hand out medals to women who don't use an epidural. As always, this is your personal choice, which you can make based on all the pros and cons below. You shouldn't be cajoled into an epidural by busy maternity staff. Similarly, if you request an epidural you should get one.

What is it?

An epidural involves painkilling drugs being passed into the small of your back via a fine tube. It is a regional anaesthetic, so the drug is injected around the nerves that carry signals from the part of your body that feels pain in labour. It will numb your tummy and provide you with very effective pain relief. In the UK, epidurals must be given by an anaesthetist. About 30 per cent of women have an epidural during labour.

Epidurals are available only in obstetrician-led maternity units. So you can't have one at a free-standing or 'alongside' **birth centre** (see page 68), or if you have a **home birth** (see page 197).

Most hospitals use low-dose epidurals that contain a mixture of painkilling drugs, usually a local anaesthetic, bupivacaine or levobupivacaine, and an opioid (fentanyl). A low-dose epidural might allow you to have some sensation in your legs and feet. A mobile epidural, which requires extra staff to monitor you, allows you to move about and keep gravity onside.

How is an epidural given?

You will sit on the edge of a bed wearing a hospital gown (if you want to) and lean forward (this is a great moment to get a cuddle from your partner and do some relaxing deep breathing). Keep as still as possible. The anaesthetist will give you a local anaesthetic in your lower back and then guide a hollow needle between the small bones in your spine.

The needle goes into the space between the layers of tissue in your spinal column (the dural space). A fine tube (catheter) is then passed through the needle and the needle is removed. The tube is taped up your back and over your shoulder. Very clever.

If you have accessed a mobile epidural, the doctors will want to check that you have sufficient sensation in your legs to move about, and you will be closely monitored.

Injection with top-ups

Painkillers are injected into the tube to numb the lower part of your tummy, and your contractions should no longer be painful. As the epidural begins to wear off, you can have top-ups, which last between one to two hours.

Continuous infusion

An epidural catheter is set up, with the other end of the tube attached to a pump. This continuously feeds the pain-relieving epidural solution into your back. You can also have stronger top-up doses of local anaesthetic, if you need them. Sometimes the pump is under your control. This is called patient-controlled epidural analgesia (PCEA) and only a minority of hospitals will not provide this. If you still have a 'breakthrough' pain that isn't being managed, the anaesthetist can give a one-off, larger dose.

Combined spinal epidural (CSE)

This injection contains a low dose of pain-relieving drugs (a mini-spinal) and works more quickly than an epidural alone. The anaesthetist will insert a catheter, and when the mini-spinal injection starts to wear off, your anaesthetist will pass the epidural solution through the tube to give you ongoing pain relief.

Checks

With all these procedures, your anaesthetist will check that your pain relief is working by using a cold spray or an ice cube on your tummy and legs, to see if you can feel it. If you can feel the coldness of the spray, your epidural may need to be adjusted or reinserted.

When is the best time to have an epidural?

You can have an epidural at any point in your labour, but most women request it when their contractions are getting strong, often when their cervix has dilated to about 5 or 6cm.

You may be offered an epidural if your labour has to be speeded up with a Syntocinon drip, because this can make your contractions intense and difficult to cope with. In this instance you can have it at any time – when as little as 2cm dilated.

Once your epidural is in place, it can stay in until after your baby is born and your placenta is delivered. It can also provide pain relief after the birth if you need stitches.

Advantages

- It's the most effective form of pain relief during labour.
- Top-ups can usually be given by an experienced midwife once the epidural is in place, meaning no waiting for an anaesthetist.
- You may still be aware of your contractions, and have a clear mind, but you'll feel no pain.
- If you have high blood pressure, it can help to lower it.
- It can be topped up with stronger local anaesthetic if you need an unplanned caesarean.

Disadvantages

- For about one woman in eight it doesn't work adequately and only numbs parts of their tummy. In this case, extra pain relief might be needed. If you're not pain-free within 30 minutes of the epidural starting, ask the anaesthetist to come back to adjust it or try again.
- Although it works fairly quickly, it takes about 20 minutes to insert and set up and another 20 minutes to work once the anaesthetic has been injected. This is longer than most other types of pain relief.
- It might make you feel shivery.

- It might cause itching, particularly if you have a CSE, but it's not usually severe.
- You may develop a fever.
- You will need to stay in bed, as your legs are likely to feel weak or heavy. Even if you are able to shuffle around on the bed, you won't be able to walk around.
- Not many hospitals offer true mobile epidurals that reduce the pain but allow you to keep mobile – ask if yours does.
- You need to keep varying the position you are sitting or lying in. This prevents you from developing a pressure sore on the numbed area of your body.
- It can affect your ability to wee, so you might need a catheter during labour or after the birth. This usually won't need to be left in, and will be used to drain your full bladder; however, if you have a difficult vaginal birth or a caesarean, you might need the catheter to be left in for longer.
- You will need more monitoring. Your baby's heartbeat will be monitored continuously for at least 30 minutes at first, and then after each top-up. Your blood pressure will be taken every 5 minutes when the epidural is started, for about 15 minutes, and after each top-up. This is because the epidural can cause your blood pressure to fall.
- You're more likely to need your labour speeded up with a Syntocinon drip; however, hospital staff should give you the chance to have a longer, slower labour, before using drugs to speed it up. Discuss this with them.
- The second stage of labour, the pushing stage, might last longer if you have an epidural. You may not feel an urge to push. If this is the case, and there's no sign of your baby's

head yet, waiting one to two hours, or until you feel the urge to push, should be encouraged.

- There's more chance of your baby needing to be born with the aid of forceps or ventouse. This may be because epidurals can make it difficult for your baby to move into the best position for birth.
- Your baby is more likely to end up in a posterior position by the time you're ready to give birth. This can happen even if he wasn't in that position when your labour started.
- There is a small risk of you having a severe headache. This can happen if the epidural needle punctures the bag of fluid that surrounds the spinal cord, causing a leak. There is about a one in 100 chance of this happening. It is usually treated by lying flat for 24–48 hours, but if it isn't resolved, you will have to go back into hospital (if you have left) to have a dural blood patch. This means taking a small amount of blood from your arm, and injecting it into your back to seal the hole made by the needle.
- There's a very small risk of nerve damage, leaving you with a numb patch on your leg or foot, or a weak leg. But this rarely happens. The risk is about 1 in 1,000 for temporary nerve damage and one in 13,000 for permanent damage.

How might an epidural affect your baby?

If your blood pressure drops, it may affect the flow of oxygen to your baby. Before starting your epidural, a small tube (intravenous cannula) will be inserted into your hand or arm. This is so that fluids and drugs can be fed through if your blood pressure falls later on.

Epidural solutions contain the opioid fentanyl, or a similar drug, which can cross the placenta. In larger doses (more than 100mg), these drugs may affect your baby's breathing, or make him drowsy. This can affect how quickly and efficiently the baby breastfeeds.

What else should you know?

The good news is that your consent will be sought for an epidural. The bad news is that your consent will be sought for an epidural – this is when you may be screaming at them to just put the paper to one side and give you the damn thing!

■ EPISIOTOMY

This is a small cut that is made to the perineum from the edge of the vagina. They should only be performed if they are absolutely necessary to make space to get a baby out or to prevent a more serious tear. The strongest clinical indication is when the baby needs to be out on the next contraction because its heartbeat indicates this to be wise. Thankfully, those instances are not as common as they used to be.

If there is time and you don't have an epidural on board, the perineum is given a small injection to numb the area so that you don't feel any pain from this little snip. Your consent will need to be sought. The cut is made at a slight diagonal away from your bottom. It takes a brief moment and the skin is normally so stretched by the baby's head that you may not feel anything. They are no longer automatically given at an assisted delivery. Midwives can give episiotomies.

You will always be stitched afterwards, as the area is very

vascular: there is a good blood supply so you can bleed heavily. But the medics will know this and get you sutured (stitched) promptly.

Recovery can be painful, so make sure you take regular anti-inflammatory ibuprofen tablets to reduce swelling. Homeopathy can be helpful at this time when other drugs are prohibited due to breastfeeding.

It is impossible to know who will or won't have an episiotomy, but perineal massage (see page 272) before birth might help the area stretch more easily, as will using more upright positions in **labour** (see page 232).

It can be really distressing to have had an episiotomy. Talk about it and don't be afraid to debrief what happened with someone you trust (see **shut up!** page 306).

ESTIMATED DATE OF DELIVERY – SEE INDUCTION (PAGE 220)

EXERCISE

After at least a decade of holding in your stomach, letting it all hang out during pregnancy can feel like Nelson Mandela did as he stepped off Robben Island after 25 years of incarceration. The temptation is to liberate your stomach muscles the moment you set down the positive pregnancy test and let your gut swing free, and boy – it can feel so good. Remember, though, however alluring it might feel to sit on the sofa feeling all squishy for the next two years, you won't enjoy your pregnancy, birth or baby if you're so unfit that you can't lift the car seat.

Unless you enter Ironman events, **labour** (see page 232) is likely to be the most physically demanding act you undertake. If you get to the delivery suite needing a water-station and a rub-down after walking from the car, it's going to be much tougher than if you arrive feeling strong, fit and with enough muscle tone to support yourself on all fours. It's pure common sense: a healthy body will increase your chances of a straightforward labour from which you will recover more quickly.

If you struggle to get motivated to exercise, consider the fact that you're now walking/swimming/doing yoga for your unborn baby. They won't thank you for it (you're about to be a mother, get used to never being thanked for anything) but when you're able to be up and about, pushing a pram and coping moderately well with sleep deprivation, they will be secretly happy.

The global expert on this topic is Professor Greg Whyte. He is a physical activity expert, world-renowned sports scientist and author of *Bump it Up: The Dynamic, Flexible Exercise and Healthy Eating Plan for Before, During and After Pregnancy*.

These are his top tips for exercising in pregnancy:

Professor Greg Whyte on exercise

Exercise should be an integral part of your life – not just during pregnancy. It leads to improvements in your physical, mental and social health while reducing many potential complications for you and your baby.

Exercise during pregnancy should be tailored to your needs and likes and should be an enjoyable part of pregnancy life. Below, I have outlined my top tips, to which there is one important caveat: these are based on a 'low-risk' pregnancy. The vast majority of pregnancies are low-risk with no pre-existing health issues. This status can change throughout pregnancy, and you should always keep in close contact with your healthcare team before starting exercise, and regularly during the nine-month period, to ensure you are exercising safely. If your pregnancy is not considered low risk, you can, and should, still exercise, but you will have to modify your programme.

How much? Your goals should be similar to those when you are not pregnant. You should aim for 30 minutes of moderate-intensity aerobic activity on most days of the week, two whole-body strength sessions per week, regular core strength and stability, and daily pelvic-floor exercises.

How hard? There are lots of ways to monitor your exercise to remain at or below a moderate intensity. Here is a simple guide:

- Rating of perceived exertion (RPE) uses a simple number scale from 0 to 10, where 0 equals sitting watching TV, to 10, which equals the hardest you have ever exercised. Your target on the RPE scale is 7.
- Using wearable tech (such as a FitBit) you can now easily monitor your heart rate. Your target throughout pregnancy should be up to 75 per cent of your maximum heart rate. Seventy-five per cent of maximum heart rate equals (220 minus your age) × 0.75.
- The 'talk test' is a great way to estimate how hard you are working. In general, during easy exercise (such as an RPE of 3–5) you are able to hold a full conversation without breaks. As the exercise moves

into the moderate territory (such as an RPE of 5–7), your conversation will be broken as your breathing rate increases, and although you will be able to talk, you won't be able to sing (which might already be true before starting exercise). During high-intensity exercise (such as an RPE of 8–10), you can only speak in short sentences or single words. So, if you're unsure whether you've hit an RPE of 7 or not, have a chat.

The exercise cycle Every session should follow the same pattern: (1) warm-up; (2) flexibility; (3) exercise; (4) cool-down. A warm-up improves your performance, reduces the potential for injury and protects your baby. Always begin an exercise session slowly, progressively increasing intensity up to the intended level for your session followed by some stretching exercises. Avoid stopping exercise abruptly; using a cool-down helps to return you to a pre-exercise state.

Stretching the limits During pregnancy you produce the hormone relaxin, which increases the laxity (flexibility) of your joints. It is important to keep up your flexibility during pregnancy, but be careful not to over-stretch. The same advice holds true for classes like yoga.

Maintenance, not improvement Exercise during pregnancy is primarily focused on maintaining your fitness over the three trimesters. Because of the changes in your body, it is unlikely that you will improve your fitness. This is why it is important to enter into pregnancy in good shape.

Moving backwards is going in the right direction
As you progress through your pregnancy, it is
important to recognise your limitations when it
comes to intensity, balance and coordination. When
it comes to exercise classes, think about moving from
advanced to intermediate to beginner as your pregnancy
progresses. Moving to lower-intensity, less-complex
classes means you can keep doing the exercise you love
safely.

Variety is the spice of life If you are finding it difficult
to complete your exercise all in one go, think about
splitting it up into smaller packages; for example, rather
than 30 minutes, you can gain the same benefits from
three lots of ten minutes' exercise. In addition, adding
something different from your exercise programme by
taking up a new exercise or joining a class can give you the
motivational boost you need.

Heating up During pregnancy your metabolism (how
much energy you produce and consume) increases, which
leads to an increased production of heat. When you add
exercise to the mix, your temperature rises more than
usual. It is important to avoid overheating during exercise,
so here are some simple tips:

- Avoid high-intensity exercise – the harder the
  exercise, the higher your temperature.
- Keep well hydrated – increased sweating can lead to
  dehydration; top up regularly during exercise.
- Clothing – wear multiple thin layers which you can
  remove as you heat up.

- Go easy in the heat – as the temperature rises, think about reducing your intensity.

Fuelling exercise During pregnancy, you will use carbohydrate at a greater rate, both at rest and during exercise, compared to when you're not pregnant. So a little extra carbohydrate in your diet won't hurt, but remember we are talking about complex carbohydrates such as potatoes, pasta, rice, and so on, not sugars, which can be problematic in excess.

A pain in the back! Ninety per cent of women experience back pain during pregnancy. Focusing on core strength and stability as well as posture (seating, standing and lying) becomes increasingly important as your bump grows.

Invisible exercise Exercising your pelvic floor during pregnancy is a must. The great thing about pelvic-floor exercises is that you can do them anytime, anywhere and no one will ever know. (See also **pelvic floor**, page 269.)

Avoid the abs As your bump grows, the stress on your abdominal muscles increases, which can cause them to stretch, leading to diastasis recti (a painless splitting of the abdominals). You should avoid exercises that focus on your abdominals, such as sit-ups, particularly during trimesters two and three. But don't be afraid to 'give your baby a hug' (slowly contracting and releasing your abs) at any time – it can help keep them strong, and it reminds you to be aware of your posture.

Take control Concentrate on technique, and maintain control throughout your exercises; never rush or make sudden and rapid changes in direction.

And breathe! Breathing is an important part of strength, and core strength and stability exercise. Make sure you concentrate on your breathing by slowly exhaling during contractions. Do not hold your breath; although this is unlikely to be a problem for your baby, it might lead to light-headedness and dizziness for you.

Don't go it alone Find a buddy to exercise with, or an antenatal class to join. Sharing your exercise makes it easier and more fun.

Every little helps Adding small amounts of activity to your everyday life can have a huge impact on your overall activity level; for example, get off the bus a stop earlier and walk the rest of the way to work, take the stairs instead of the lift or walk to the shops rather than drive.

It's never too late You can begin exercising at any stage of pregnancy, so never think you've left it too late. As long as you remember to start easy and progress slowly, listening to your body throughout, and remain at or below an RPE of 7 (75 per cent of your maximum heart rate), you'll be able to enjoy the benefits of exercise whenever you start. And, if nothing else, you can do your pelvic-floor exercises anywhere and at any time.

Enjoy it Exercise should be fun, not a chore. It is not uncommon to feel too tired to exercise at times during pregnancy; however, a gentle exercise session, no matter how short, can help ease those aches and pains without too much effort. In addition, completing a session will make you feel like you are doing something positive to help yourself, which will make you feel a whole lot better.

F is for ...

FEAR

It's widely recognised within the birth community that we are in the midst of a global pandemic of fear surrounding birth. Women must always have possessed some trepidation towards bringing a new life into the world. It's a massive responsibility, and the sheer physics of getting '*that* out of *that*' seems insane, despite the fact that human beings (as we know them) have been managing to reproduce for 200,000 years.

Ironically, as birth has become more medicalised, with the intention of making the process safer, it has also become more frightening. This was never the aim of medical professionals (unless you live in Brazil, where common tales of women being bullied in labour and enforced caesareans will stop you in your tracks). But a consequence of hospitalising such a large majority of births is that it has become shut away, sanitised and kept out of the sight of young women. As with everything in life, the unknown is eminently more frightening than the reality.

Instead, we have our pick of dramatic, media-based births that allow directors to use their things-are-going-wrong music, and labour is used to signpost pain, terror, blood and near, or in some particularly disturbing scenes actual, death. It really is no wonder that more and more women are spending 40 weeks of pregnancy with their legs crossed wondering how the hell they are going to survive that shit. It takes a fierce mentality to keep those images from seeping into your mind and locking your cervix perfectly shut.

Don't be surprised, then, if you are frightened of labour. That's (sadly) completely normal these days, but there is a lot that you can do to alleviate your anxieties: talk through your feelings with a **Hypnobirthing** coach (see page 206) who can help you to dissolve them; seek out the best medical support you can afford so that you have continuity of care in your pregnancy and labour; join an antenatal course that will empower you with knowledge and positivity.

Disconnect from fear

When other women launch into a terrifying tale of a friend of a friend who had an awful birth, politely state that it's not helpful for you to hear that with labour around the corner, and change the subject. Or, put your fingers in your ears and shout, 'La! La! La! I'm not listening to your awful story, you psychotic torturer!' The approach you choose will largely depend on how well you know this person and whether you intend to remain friends.

If you think you might be suffering from tokophobia – a genuine, debilitating fear of labour (this actually keeps some women from ever falling pregnant) – talk to your care providers. Tokophobic women may be able to access therapeutic mental-health services, which will often take them on a fascinating journey to uncover the seed of their anxiety. They may offer cognitive behavioural therapy to consciously challenge your preconceptions, or hypnosis to clear out the negative blockages at the back of the mind. It is also completely reasonable to ask for a **caesarean birth** (see page 115) in these circumstances.

Maggie Howell created Natal Hypnotherapy and birthed her five boys at home. Here are her insights:

Maggie Howell on Hynotherapy and birth

Over the last 15 years I have worked with hundreds of women, and in over 80 per cent of cases fear is the main emotion that they associate with birth. Simple biology and clinical evidence proves that if fear is present in a labouring woman, her experience will be more painful and challenging.

Imagine yourself labouring in a jungle. You suddenly see, or even think you see, a wild animal lurking in the shadows. What would happen? Would you have a conscious choice on what happens next? You might think you could control the situation, but your body would already have made the decision.

Simply believing there is a wild animal in your birth space would instantly stimulate a healthy fight-or-flight mechanism. Labour contractions would slow down or stop and would not resume until you felt safe.

This fear activates the nervous system to produce adrenalin (the danger hormone), which gives you the oomph or power to prepare to fight or to run away. Your cervix tightens (to prevent your baby from being born where it is not safe) and the increased level of adrenalin neutralises the oxytocin (the hormone responsible for stimulating your uterus to contract) and endorphins (the pain-killing hormone), so that the body naturally slows down or even stops birthing. Experiencing fear during labour leads to your heat rate increasing, your breathing becoming shallow and faster (so reducing the amount of oxygen in your body and your baby), your heart pumping blood faster around your body, so raising your blood pressure and directing blood away from your uterus (and your baby) to your limbs, to prepare you for action.

All this fight-or-flight preparation uses a great deal of energy. As our bodies were only designed to be in this heightened sense of preparation to fight or flight for a few minutes at a time, you can imagine that staying in this state for prolonged periods of time will be extremely draining, if not dangerous.

You might be asking, 'What does a woman giving birth in a jungle have to do with me?' Well, it is more about the fear than the location: fear of pain, fear of dying, fear of tearing, fear of losing control. Your nervous system does not know the difference between real or imagined danger or fear, and so it will respond in the same way to both.

The effects of fear vs relaxation on you and your baby
If you go into birth feeling and being frightened, your system will respond accordingly. This fear will lead to increased adrenalin in your body, leading to increased tension in your muscles and your cervix. Less contraction hormones will be produced so that your uterus is having to work much harder to flex and tighten. This subsequently makes contractions far more painful, in the same way that if you tense up when you are in pain, the pain becomes far greater.

How, then, does being relaxed and calm, rather than fearful and tense, make a difference?

By being relaxed during your labour, your body responds in a very different way to the fear scenario described above. When you are relaxed, your breathing is even and rhythmical, ensuring a high level of oxygen is entering your body. This oxygen goes through to your baby, ensuring that your baby remains calm and stable. Increased oxygen stimulates the production of oxytocin and endorphins. Your blood pressure remains at a healthy level, and, as your body is limp and relaxed, you conserve your energy, with all the excess energy being channelled through to the muscle that is really working hard, namely your uterus. As the uterus has no resistance or tension from surrounding muscles, the contractions are more effective and more comfortable. As the labour progresses unhindered by artificial hormones, other natural hormones kick in, including relaxin, which allows the cells of the birth canal to relax, soften and stretch, so making the baby's descent easier and more comfortable.

How do you decrease fear and increase a sense of calm?

I was recently watching a Will Smith movie, *After Earth*, and heard this fantastic quote: 'Fear is not real. It is a product of our imagination, causing us to fear things that do not at present and may not ever exist. Do not misunderstand me, danger is very real, but fear is a choice.'

Always remember that 'fear is not real' and 'fear is a choice'. At any given time you can make a choice to stop being scared about something that may or may not happen in the future. Just because your aunt had a terrible birth, or the c-section rate at your hospital is high or you've binge-watched *One Born Every Minute*, it does not mean that those experiences have to become your experience.

What should you do if a fear or worry crops up? Well, following this ABCD method is a great start:

A. **Acknowledge and accept it** Simply tell a friend about it, or write it down, type up your fears, or draw a picture showing your fears, then . . .

B. **Banish it** Burn the paper, or delete the document word by word, imagine dropping your fears down a well, scrunch up the drawing, then stop everything and . . .

C. **Connect with the here and now** Take a few deep breaths, feel your shoulders drop, relax your hands and focus on the amazing ability of your body to grow a baby. Notice where you are right now, and then . . .

D. **Disassociate and let it go** Actively give yourself a good talking to and step away from the fear. Worrying about it now will not change anything – it just wastes a lot of valuable emotional and mental energy.

By following the above steps, the fear is no longer able to fester and grow out of proportion to your reality right now.

Another great way to get rid of fears and to learn to be more relaxed, calm and in control is to listen to a Hypnotherapy recording (see **Hypnobirthing**, page 206, for more on this).

Women have been giving birth for millennia. There is nothing to fear.

FORMULA AND BOTTLE FEEDING

Thanks to the extremely skilful way that formula-milk companies surreptitiously market their wares, it is easy to think that formula milk is as good (if not better) for your baby than breast milk. This is not true. **Breastfeeding** (see page 78) has countless benefits for the health of your baby and also for you. Milk-formula companies are very clever at stealth marketing and have done a great job of portraying their products as equal to – or better than – your own.

Nevertheless, for women who wish to breastfeed but aren't supported to do so, those who choose not to breastfeed at all, those who eventually move onto formula, or those who combine both types, formula milk is the ticket to happily enjoying their babies.

The kit

You don't need to buy all the formula kit and caboodle before your baby arrives, but if you do find the time is right to formula feed, this is what you will need.

Milk

Formula feeding with powder will cost you roughly £10 per week (plus the initial outlay for bottles and a steriliser). The ready-made cartons are much more expensive. Newborn formula is the only type that is appropriate for your new baby.

Formula is usually made from cow's milk that has been treated to make it suitable for babies and contains whey protein. Your baby can stay on this alone until they are six months old (unless your doctor has, for some reason, suggested otherwise). It's also suitable once you introduce solid foods (at about six months) and can be used up to 12 months of age.

There is no evidence that one brand of infant formula is any better or worse than any other. But if you suspect a particular brand disagrees with your baby, try another. Your health visitor should be able to discuss this with you.

Please ignore ridiculous labels about formula milk for 'hungrier babies', 'follow on' or 'night time'. This marketing simply plays on new mums' fears that they may be depriving their ravenous child; it gets them to part with more of their hard-earned cash and manipulates their sleep-deprived mind into believing that their child will sleep 7/7 if only it wasn't hungry! These milks can be harmful to babies under six months old and yet the labelling is not always clear – buy carefully.

Other types of formula

Soya infant formula is made from soya beans rather than cow's milk. Don't use this unless it has been prescribed or recommended by your GP. If your baby is diagnosed as being allergic to cow's milk, your GP will prescribe an appropriate infant formula with fully hydrolysed proteins. Infant formula with partially hydrolysed proteins is available in the shops, but this is not suitable for babies with a cow's milk allergy.

Goat's milk-based formula is produced to the same nutritional standards as cow's milk-based formula. These are unsuitable for infants with a cow's milk protein allergy and should not be given to them, unless recommended by a health professional.

Remember, if you have any questions about the infant formula you are giving your baby, you can ask your local pharmacist, midwife, health visitor or GP.

Bottles

Whether you are using formula or expressed breast milk, you will need to buy several bottles, teats and lids. As everything must be fully sterilised before use, the number of bottles you need will probably be related to how organised you are. It's easy to forget when you arrive home after a day out, that there are three used bottles in the bottom of your nappy changing bag and two dirty ones in the dishwasher. This is normally the point at which your baby will start crying for his tea!

There's no evidence that one type of teat or bottle is better than any other, but look for ones that most mirror a female nipple. Midwives with a knowledge of breastfeeding tend to recommend Nuk. You might even notice that your baby prefers one type to another. But stick with them for a few days at least before you spend more money.

It's important to wash out bottles with washing up liquid and a 'special' (as in, just for this purpose as opposed to extraordinary) bottle brush. You can also stick them in the dishwasher, of course, but check that any dried-on milk has been fully removed before you use them. You can turn the teats inside out before you put them in the dishwasher.

Be prepared for the fact that losing bottle lids will become a constant source of frustration and bewilderment. It is entirely possible to leave the house with three and return with only one. And it's possible to do this every single day for a year – or at least it would be if they were easier to buy. Some brands only sell replacement bottle lids if you buy the whole kit and caboodle again. These manufacturers are evil. I believe there is a thief who lives on a plastic island in the Atlantic built entirely from bottle lids. And he's laughing at our forgetful stupidity.

Sterilisers

These will become the third person in your relationship for at least six months. Read the instructions with your partner at a time when you won't be distracted by a crying baby. You will find that no matter how many masters degrees you and your partner hold between you, baby-based equipment will demand a far greater level of education, ingenuity and perseverance than your pre-baby life ever required.

Oh, and do yourself a favour: make sure you aren't the only person in the house who knows how to use the steriliser. Dads are great at this shit – it's the combination of mechanical kit, straightforward instructions and echoes of steam engines. Plus, most dads really want to help. So, if you are still on maternity leave, consider setting him the job of filling the bottles with boiled, chilled water before he goes to work for the day. And silently thank him every three to four hours.

Electric steam sterilisers Sterilisers are much less hassle than they were a few years ago (and much easier than boiling equipment in cauldrons, as our mothers had to do). There are various types of steriliser to suit all tastes and budgets. If you're a frequent steriliser, zapping milky germs from dawn till dusk, you probably want the electric steam type that, once plugged into the mains will produce six bottles and teats within six to eight minutes. Before you were a mum, that was the length of time you would spend painting individual fingernails. Once you have a baby, six to eight minutes is the window in which you will put on a white wash, empty a nappy bin and make a sandwich (that you will forget to eat). These sterilisers are the most expensive and will take up space on your kitchen work surface, but they're worth it for the convenience of sterilising a whole day's worth of bottles in one go while also timing your Billy Whizz moves around the kitchen.

Microwave sterilisers are more affordable and won't clutter up your kitchen. They're also the speediest version, usually taking about three minutes in the microwave; however, this is still time to go to the loo, move that box of crap from the bottom of the stairs and conduct one round of the muslin-pick-up steeplechase around the lounge. Microwave sterilisers are compact enough to store in a cupboard and take with you when you're travelling. The main drawback is that they don't hold as much feeding kit in one go as an electric steam steriliser, but if you're happy to sterilise little and often, they're a smart buy.

Self-sterilising bottles or disposable steriliser bags If your baby is mostly breastfed and you only need to sterilise very occasionally, self-sterilising bottles or disposable steriliser bags could be a better option than buying a proper steriliser. Both types work in the microwave: steriliser bags generally hold one or two bottles or a breast pump, whereas steriliser bottles sterilise themselves. They're great for travelling and are easy to store.

Sterilising tablets Believe it or not, hospitals use old-fashioned water-based steriliser on the postnatal wards – simply leaving the bottles and so on in a bowl of cold water with sterilising tablets. Very 1972. But it's certainly cheap, and many women still find the simplicity very appealing

How to bottle feed

Find yourself a comfortable spot and pick up your baby. Yes, I did just patronise you. But, for the love of God, look around any coffee shop and you will see adults holding a bottle in the mouth of a baby which is still strapped in a car seat or pram while mum/dad/carer looks at their phone or chats to their friend. This is not cool. It's the equivalent of being forced to eat alone at your desk without even being able to read the showbiz section on the *Daily*

Mail website. Your baby wants to be held. Your baby *needs* to be held! They want to look into their carer's eyes, hear their voice and see a smiling face.

Also, consider the position of a baby's gut if they are in a car seat or baby carrier – they aren't relaxed, upright or able to squirm about. Put yourself in their shoes as much as you can. Would you want to eat your lunch in a semi-reclined, over-the-shoulder rollercoaster seat, even if you were stationary? So, hold your baby, snuggled up against you and keep them fairly upright for bottle feeds.

Support your baby's head so that they can breathe and swallow comfortably. Brush the teat against their lips and, when they open their mouth wide, let them draw in the teat. It's vital to keep the teat full of milk. If you can see any air space inside the teat, it is likely to be ingested and come back to haunt your baby as painful wind and you will drown in vomit.

Bottle-fed babies are much windier than breastfed babies. This is partly because the milk is taken on board more quickly, at a pace they have less control over. If you've ever experienced the dentist's chair vodka game, you'll know what I'm talking about.

Unless your baby is crying hysterically (in which case, removing the bottle might result in more wind), try giving her a couple of minutes of milk before taking her off for a quick winding. Hold her against your chest so that her face is looking over your shoulder, or hold her upright on your knee with one hand under her chin and the other hand completely flat against her spine. The key is to give her a straight back and therefore windpipe (think about the way your husband so pleasingly straightens up to get rid of a satisfying belch). After baby has surprised herself with a lovely little burpy-pops (insert own cute word here), continue feeding. If a baby takes a whole feed with wind beneath the milk, she is more likely to bring lots of it back up again. This is bloody annoying. It will keep your washing machine on permanently, and ten years from now you'll find yourself absent-mindedly scraping a five-pence-piece-sized dry sick patch off your sofa.

When baby is sick

Some babies are just more sicky than others. You'll soon get to know your own baby and wonder what life was like before you were cocooned by bibs and muslins.

Of course, it can be shocking and upsetting when your baby is sick. I've heard of some poor couples rushing their newborn off to A&E as they thought such positing was evidence that he was seriously ill.

It's also immensely disheartening when your baby suddenly brings up every last ounce of milk you just spent 40 minutes lovingly providing. If you weren't already on the verge of tears, you will be now. But, don't worry, they probably kept down more than you realise. Try winding him at the start of a feed (as above). Also, consider whether you might be over-feeding him. Babies' bodies are sensitive: if there is too much milk to digest in a single feed, they will let you know. Check that the hole in your baby's teat is not too big – giving milk too quickly can cause sickness. Sitting your baby upright on your lap after a feed may help. Similarly, the teat shouldn't be too small, as your baby will have to work so hard to get the milk out that they eventually get tired and give up, waking up a little while later still hungry. Also, it can be really easy to forget that you are still using newborn teats when the baby is a few months old.

In order to avoid this gulping-and-vomiting pattern, always give your baby plenty of time to feed without being rushed. This isn't always easy, especially if you have older children, but it will make the whole experience of motherhood less fraught if you can forward plan a tad and use feeding time to just chill the heck out.

If your baby brings up a lot of milk, they may be hungry again sooner than usual. But don't be tempted to force them to take more milk than they want during a feed just to spread them out.

If your baby is sick repeatedly, isn't producing plenty of wet nappies and appears to be in pain, talk to your health visitor or GP.

How much formula do I need to feed a newborn baby?

This is extremely difficult to answer, as each baby is different: some will prefer snacking little and often, and some will take a full tummy and remain satisfied for two to three hours. Even children born to the same mum will have different habits. But remember that newborn tummies are absolutely tiny: roughly the size of a large marble. They can only take approximately 5ml per feed (a typical baby's bottle holds 250ml) so never force a baby to finish a bottle. They are developing a reflex that tells them when they are full – let this evolve.

Offer your baby some milk when they appear hungry: when they are turning their head sideways, routing around for a teat and crying. But be careful not to mistake tiredness for hunger. Tired babies will often cry when they want to sleep. Ask yourself when they last fed and how much they had. Could it be that they just want a cuddle and to fall asleep on your chest?

As tempting as it might be when you want to renew the car insurance or make the bed, never leave a baby alone to feed with a propped-up bottle. No chore is so important that you risk your baby choking on their milk.

Talk to your health visitor or other mothers with experience of bottle feeding, if you need help. You'll find the phone number for your health visitor in your baby's **Red Book** (see page 300).

How do I make up formula milk?

To make up a bottle of powdered formula, follow the instructions on the packet carefully. Here's my idiot's guide:

1. Sterilise bottle, teat and lid.
2. Boil tap water and pour the exact amount into the bottle. Leave it to cool until it is warm.
3. Add the right number of scoops to the bottle with the scoop provided, using a clean knife to level it off.
4. Put on the teat and cover, and give the bottle a good shake until all the powder has dissolved.
5. Test the temperature by tipping a little milk out of the teat on to the inside of your wrist. It should feel just warm, not hot.

The temperature of the milk is important: too cold from the fridge and your baby may recoil. Too hot and you might burn them. Rather than obsessing about heating and cooling, you may want to partly fill the bottles with boiled water in the morning; place them in the fridge and simply top up to the correct, safe temperature with freshly boiled water at feeding time. Always shake well and check the temperature on your hand.

For about £70 you can now buy a machine that makes up bottles to the exact temperature in two minutes. Think of it as the baby's own cappuccino machine. It takes up space in your kitchen but certainly helps with speeding up your pace of life.

Can I make up a feed to store in the fridge for later?

Ideally not, as milk powder isn't sterile, and bacteria may survive in it. Having said that, there may be times when you need to make up a feed in advance; for example, if you have twins, or if you're out shopping and you don't want to make a feed where there are lots of bacteria around. It's best to prepare just one feed for later use. You can do this as safely as possible by putting the feed in the fridge or a cool bag as soon as you've made it. Use it within four hours if it's been stored in a cool bag, or within 12 hours if it's been in the fridge.

My baby is fed, so why is he now so grumpy?

If your baby swallows air while bottle feeding and is quickly put down to sleep, he may feel uncomfortable and cry. Remember the wedding buffets at which you've eaten too much after three weeks of dieting? Well, it's a bit like that, and babies don't even have our developed gut. So after a feed, try not to lay them down straight away. Hold your baby upright against a shoulder (even if they fell asleep on the bottle) and gently rub their back; any trapped air can find its way out easily, and milk can be digested with gravity's helping hand before you lie them down.

Of course, what goes in must come out, so you will find that your baby commonly does a poo during or after a feed. You'll get to know their habits and will soon become adept at nappy-change timing: why bother with a fresh one just before a feed when you know he is about to fill it?

Could formula feeding make my baby constipated?

Despite the fact that you will often lose count due to fatigue, distractions or a wandering mind (who knew counting to five was so hard?), always use the recommended amount of powder scoops stated on the packet. Don't add extra formula to fill them up. Too much can make your baby constipated and may cause dehydration.

If your baby is under eight weeks old and hasn't had a poo for two to three days, discuss this with your midwife, health visitor or GP, particularly if they're gaining weight slowly (the baby, not the GP). Your baby should be growing and having plenty of wet and dirty nappies.

FREEBIRTHING

I know this is an era in which all choices must be respected and every woman has the right to birth wherever she wants and with whom. I totally subscribe to that enlightened view. But if you are considering freebirthing, that is, giving birth alone, without a medical attendant present – I have only one question: ARE YOU BLOODY MAD??!

Sadly, freebirthing is on the rise. Why? Because women have crappy first births and don't want to risk another one. But instead of fighting for a one-to-one midwife or prioritising/raising funds to hire one, more and more women are choosing to birth alone – normally at home – without anyone present except, perhaps, their partner.

I can hear you gasping at how dangerous this must be and how stupid they are to risk the well-being of their child. But it's more nuanced than that. The motivation for freebirthing is normally quite the opposite: these women believe that hospitals are a bit quick to administer unnecessary procedures that can cause harm to them or their babies. And they are right. But having a home birth with a medically qualified midwife in the house is very different from going it alone. So far, there have been no incidences of freebirths going wrong or babies being harmed, so we shouldn't be too alarmed.

If the numbers increase, however, it is possible – but not inevitable – that babies will be affected. It's most heartbreaking of all that women are putting themselves and their babies at risk by taking themselves out of a system that they simply do not trust.

If you are tempted by freebirthing, talk through your fears and past experiences with the lead midwife in your area, and see if there is any way your requirements can be accommodated. It may be that you can have a **home birth** (see page 197) with the agreement that the midwives remain in another room, only entering intermittently to monitor and check that you are OK.

Birth is a beautiful, incredible moment of joy. It is always improved by the presence of a kind, experienced and discreet birth attendant.

G is for ...

GAS AND AIR

If I had my way, every kitchen in the land would have a handy little canister of this magic gas attached to the wall for times when mummy is feeling immensely stressed. I'm sure my husband and children would agree.

Otherwise known as entonox, it is a medical gas mixture consisting of 50 per cent nitrous oxide and 50 per cent oxygen. It's brilliant in situations where pain relief needs to be quick to begin – and quick to wear off. If you've ever dislocated a shoulder or broken a bone, you probably had a toke on gas and air to take the edge off your discomfort. Unlike an effective epidural, it won't stop the pain, but it certainly reduces the intensity and helps you to relax. (If you're still unconvinced about its effectiveness, consider that American drug companies won't allow gas and air to be offered on labour wards because it is so effective in reducing epidural use.)

It is breathed in via a plastic mouthpiece attached to a pipe. One of the best aspects of this drug is that you are in charge and choose when to inhale. It is designed for use at any stage during labour and it can be very effective towards the end of labour when pushing begins.

It is possible to overdose on gas and air and experience the sort of white-out usually associated with extreme dope-smokers. But this is not really a laughing matter; if you do pass out, lots of doctors will run in to wake you up, and your partner will forever take the piss out of you for being such a lightweight.

Tips for using gas and air

- Hold off until you absolutely need pain relief, particularly if you intend to avoid an epidural. Go too early on the G&A in labour and you might find that you need something stronger later. If you can wait until the pushing stage, G&A is likely to get you through to the end.
- Breathe deeply and slowly. Do not take short, snatched

breaths, as it will not be very effective and may make you feel dizzy.

- Take the mouthpiece out as a contraction ends, and let your jaw loosen.
- In the space between contractions, you will not need to use it.
- When you feel a contraction about to begin, place the mouthpiece in and take one long, slow breath, breathing out through your nose and mouth with the plastic loosely between your teeth. You may find each contraction uses two or three deep breaths.
- If you time the inhalations correctly, the drug will have a maximum effect at the peak of the contraction.

GENETIC TESTING

Chorionic villus sampling (CVS) is a procedure that helps to detect genetic abnormalities including Down's syndrome, Edward's syndrome, Patau's or sickle cell anaemia and has superseded the traditional amniocentesis test that can only be performed after 16 weeks of pregnancy (the insertion of a needle through the belly to extract amniotic fluid). Instead of taking a sample of **amniotic fluid** (see page 32), the CVS test removes a small sample of cells from the placenta, which can then be tested.

It's only offered if there's a high risk that your baby could have a genetic condition due to family history (for example, cystic fibrosis) or if an abnormality has been detected in a scan. You don't have to have CVS if it's offered. It's up to you to decide whether you want it. Discuss the pros and cons with your doctor. The risk of miscarriage is slightly higher than that of an amniocentesis at about 1–2 per cent; however, the benefit is that it can be performed earlier in your pregnancy: between the eleventh and fourteenth week, so you'll have more time to consider your options. The NHS is normally outstanding at handling these kinds of complex cases, and a specialist will help you consider all your choices.

GOWNGATE

A maternity morality tale – true story:

Setting: delivery suite in a busy London hospital.

Characters: pregnant woman arrives in hospital for induction. Husband. Midwife.

MIDWIFE: [reaching for a backless hospital gown]: Here is the gown you have to wear.

WOMAN: [wearing comfortable, loose clothing]: I'm actually pretty comfortable. I'd rather wear my own clothes.

MIDWIFE: You have to wear this.

WOMAN: Why?

MIDWIFE: It's hospital protocol. [Leaves room]

HUSBAND: Maybe you should wear it.

WOMAN: No! I'm not having my arse hanging out as I walk down the corridor. And why would I want to feel like a 'patient'?

[Midwife enters.]

MIDWIFE: Do you need help putting the gown on?

WOMAN: No, I'm fine wearing this.

MIDWIFE: I'll give you a few more minutes to put it on.
   [Leaves]

[HUSBAND looks open-mouthed at wife.]

[WOMAN stands and puts gown back in cupboard. Midwife

enters. Looks woman up and down, gets gown out of
wardrobe, puts it on the bed in silence and walks out.]

Fortunately, the midwifery shift changed and the next midwife
did not insist that the woman put the gown on.

Moral to the story: don't accept being treated like a child. You can
wear whatever you want in labour.

▪ GUILT

There's a very good chance that until you have a baby you do
not know what true guilt feels like. Yes, you might feel a little
disappointed in yourself after eating a whole bag of sea salt and
black pepper kettle chips with two pots of hummus for dinner,
or that texting your mum on her birthday didn't entirely assuage
the discomfort of forgetting a card (although it did a bit). But, true,
lung-emptying, bone-crushing guilt is reserved for those living
in da hood of mothers.

It wasn't always like this. Previous generations would wrap
their young in a blanket, put them in a pram at the bottom of
the garden and smoke a cigarette with their morning coffee.
As recently as the 1970s, they'd place said baby (if the foxes
hadn't eaten it) on the back seat of the car in a carrycot and
drive to the local shop. There, they'd buy tinned vegetables
and white bread, which they'd feed to elder siblings without
any over-riding concern for their nutritional needs or potential
intolerances.

Parental guilt is new. Very new. It happened when 'parenting'
became a verb in the late 1970s and early 1980s so that companies
could sell us stuff (remember you can fail at a doing word; you

can't fail at being a person, place or thing). Before that, human beings were just parents – nouns – unless it was Friday night, of course, and then they dropped that moniker to become themselves again and drank lager in the pub while you sat outside in the car.

Remember this when you feel swamped and overwhelmed that you're doing it all wrong, that your birth plan went tits up, that your 'sleep training' isn't working, and that everyone else seems to remember to put tampons in but you keep forgetting.

When it comes to being a mum, my advice is this: Lower. Your. Expectations. Babies and children need very little: warmth, food, language, love and (relatively) happy parent(s). That's it. Everything else is just icing.

When my son was about two, I went through a stage of thinking I was wetting my pants. I'd notice, every now and then, that my knickers were inexplicably wet and presumed I must have had some pelvic-floor issue. But I'd remained pretty trampoline-friendly in that department, so it didn't make sense. This went on for a few months until one day it struck me: I was forever in such a rush to go to the loo that I wasn't always pulling my own pants down far enough and thereby peeing in them. Oh, yeah – that was a proud moment: while potty training my son I needed lessons of my own. So, when I say Lower. Your. Expectations, I mean really low: eat, drink, breathe, be kind to yourself and don't piss in your own pants.

H is for ...

HAIR

Normally, we shed 50 head hairs a day (a high five to the scientist who discovered this with such accuracy). This is why, every six to eight weeks, you forget to buy drain unblocker and paddle in the shower tray. But one of the many gifts of pregnancy is that your body clings on to these 50-hairs-a-day for 40 weeks. That's 140,000 hairs on your head rather than in the plughole. This explains the glossy mane that renders pregnant women so beautiful that fathers-to-be don't run for the hills.

The bad news is that when your hormones return to normal (ha!) all this hair must surrender to the hairbrush or the plughole. Be prepared, it's quite a shock. For most women it happens three to four months after your baby is born. It's a bit rubbish, but for a while you will simply have to accept it.

Annoyingly, it also happens at a time when you may not feel terribly happy about your post-baby body; you're wearing part-maternity and part pre-baby clothes (and don't want to waste money on new ones yet) and sleep deprivation is being no ally to your skin. So, in other words, you might look in the mirror and see a fat, balding, spotty, baggy-eyed caricature of your former self. Guess what? Your baby does not see that. They see the person in the world that they love and need more than anyone else. You, being you is all they want. Everything else will come back to you in time – I promise. Even your hair will eventually grow back.

In the meantime, swish those locks with joy – because you're worth it.

HEALTH VISITOR

A health visitor is one of the many medical practitioners that you will probably never have encountered before you have a baby. Health visitors (HVs) are qualified nurses or midwives who have undergone further training in public-health nursing, with a particular emphasis on families with children under five years old. Just like any health professional, some are good, some are less so. The beauty of an HV is that they come to you. In a time when the NHS is under ever-increasing pressure, this really is a gift, so put the kettle on and pick their brains. If you are concerned that your HV has given you poor advice, seek a second opinion from your GP or midwife. But don't take it from me, listen to Vanessa Christie, herself a lactation consultant and health visitor.

Vanessa Christie on health visitors

I began my professional life as a children's nurse in the UK and then with the humanitarian medical aid agency MSF, in South Sudan. With my feet back on the ground, I quickly realised that I wanted to help keep all these little people out of hospital in the first place, so my life took a different turn.

And that's what HVs aim to do: to support you to be the best parent you can be, so that you and your children are as happy and as healthy as possible. There is no perfect way. Our aim is not to snoop around your house and hope to find it sparkling clean, with all the ironing done, fresh bread being baked, a snoozing baby settled in their basket and a fully dressed and perfectly made-up mother.

No. We don't do snooping and, in fact, we'd worry more if everything did seem too La La Land perfect.

Whether it's queries around sleep and settling, breastfeeding, bottle feeding, immunisations, bonding, colic, minor ailments, development, dental health, accident prevention, starting solid foods, behaviour management, your emotional well-being, relationship difficulties, financial worries or much more besides, the HV is your go-to listening ear and answer book for expert advice, on all things family-related, right up until your child starts school.

Frequency of visits

The HV service is fairly stretched in this day and age, and the number of times you can expect to see your HV will vary, depending on where you live in the UK and your own individual circumstances and potential needs.

Most areas aim to contact parents at least once during the pregnancy to introduce themselves and their service and to assess whether you will benefit from any enhanced support once the baby is born, for any health or social reasons.

You can then expect your HV to arrange to see you at home about 10–14 days post-delivery, which is normally the time when you are discharged from midwifery care, if all is going well. Once you know when to expect your HV's visit, it can be a good idea to put a few thoughts and questions down on paper, so that you can be confident you've covered anything that's on your mind, before she walks out of the door.

After this visit, it really does depend on where you are and what your needs are, as to how much contact you will have. As a result, don't always expect them to be checking up on you (outside the mandatory contacts they are commissioned to provide). If you feel you need further support, pick up the phone (or ask your partner or a friend to do it for you) to arrange another home visit, or just turn up at a well-baby clinic, which are drop-in sessions held on a fairly regular basis at your GP surgery or children's centre.

There are many outstanding HVs who have dedicated their lives to working with the families in their caseloads, so how do you know if you've bagged a goodie?

1. Being a new mother is a particularly vulnerable time in our lives, and any thoughts or feelings you have, positive or otherwise, are entirely valid and understandable. Your HV should make you feel relaxed, be easy to talk to and never, ever make you feel that you're being judged. She is the perfect person to off-load on to and she expects it, so go right ahead.

2. She will never utter the fateful words that 'you'll be making a rod for your own back' and will fully encourage you to listen to your instincts and support your choices to snuggle your baby and meet their needs, any time it feels right to you.

3. She will support your feeding choices, whatever they are. If you have decided you'd like to breastfeed but it turns out to be difficult at first, do make sure that either she is able to give you some top-quality support to get things going in the right direction, or refers you to a breastfeeding specialist (such as a certified lactation consultant). With the right

support, giving your baby formula if you don't
want to is much less necessary than we are led to
believe. So don't be cajoled into anything you aren't
comfortable with, without making sure it is entirely
necessary first.

4. If your baby is generally happy, healthy and
   thriving, a good HV won't make a fuss of any night
   waking – that is, unless it is a problem for you and
   you are asking for her support. You are not 'doing it
   wrong' if your baby wakes every few hours at night
   (on the contrary, this is normal baby behaviour)
   but, when you and your baby are ready, there are
   always gentle and age-appropriate methods you
   can employ to gradually help settle them for longer
   periods. Ditto the final sentence of point number 3
   above.

HEARTBURN

This is another of pregnancy's irritations and can feel like you've
just necked a litre of petrol. Hormones are to blame again,
because progesterone relaxes the sphincter at the top of your
stomach causing stomach acid to rise up into your oesophagus.
At the same time, your uterus is pressing on your diaphragm and
your stomach, making it easier for this burning fluid to rise up and
have you reaching to knock back the Gaviscon or the Rennies.
You can, of course, get such treatments *free* on prescription – you
are pregnant and have paid your taxes, so make the most of it.

Making sure you eat little but often might help to stop the
severity, and if you eat your evening meal too close to bedtime you
might find that it worsens when you lie flat. So try to eat earlier

in the evening than you normally might. You might notice that some foods make it worse: spicy dishes and citric or acidic foods are common enemies of the heartburn sufferer.

If you struggle with heartburn at night, try using extra pillows to keep you slightly upright.

Rest assured that it will stop almost as soon as your baby is out – and you will quickly forget that you ever suffered from it.

HOME BIRTH

We all love a little eavesdropping, so take a moment to listen to this conversation between a woman planning a home birth and, well – almost anyone.

HOSPITAL BIRTHER: Wow! A home birth? You're brave!

HOME BIRTHER: [shrugging] Not really . . .

HOSPITAL BIRTHER: But isn't that dangerous?

HOME BIRTHER: I've looked at the facts and decided it's not.

HOSPITAL BIRTHER: I think you're mad. How will you handle the pain?

HOME BIRTHER: I'm not sure yet. I've got a few techniques to use.

HOSPITAL BIRTHER: Well, my husband wouldn't let me do that. He'd say it's too dangerous for us both, and we really wanted this baby.

HOME BIRTHER: [patiently] We really want this baby too. I'd just feel safer at home. We'll have a midwife with us at all times and we'll transfer to hospital if we need to.

HOSPITAL BIRTHER: Then why not just start there?

HOME BIRTHER: Because I'm not ill – I don't feel I need to be in a hospital.

HOSPITAL BIRTHER: But you might *be* ill during the birth – and then what?

HOME BIRTHER: As I say, I'm happy to transfer to hospital if we have to.

HOSPITAL BIRTHER: But what about the mess! Oh my God! Imagine the blood everywhere!

HOME BIRTHER: The midwives take care of any 'mess' – and it's not like the movies, you know …

HOSPITAL BIRTHER: Everyone I know who tried to have a home birth failed, and just think of the cost to the NHS of ambulances rescuing women from failed home births.

HOME BIRTHER: I don't like the word 'failed' used about any woman who has given birth. I also think that if we use ambulances to pick hammered people off the streets at weekends we can use them for labouring women. Now would you like more coffee – or to just *sod off*?

I never fail to be amazed by how women who choose home birth are considered reckless and selfish, and are accused of putting their own experience over the safety of their baby (as a fun exercise, repeat the conversation above, swapping the home birther for a woman opting for a c-section and consider how outraged you'd be). Perhaps this fear of being judged is why celebrities who have home-birthed don't publicise the fact. Pamela Anderson, Meryl Streep, Ricki Lake, Julianne Moore, Demi Moore and Cindy Crawford are all home birthers.

Women who choose home birth are not 'brave' – the repeated use of this word always makes me smile (when I say 'smile' I mean knock back tequila shots and bang my head on the table to numb the frustration). 'Brave' people do risky things; 'brave' people have white knuckles as they venture into the potentially death-defying unknown; brave people don't use tea-lights to prettify a room and laugh with a committed midwife as their partner fills the birth pool.

For the vast majority of women, a home birth is completely devoid of drama or fear.

In 2015 The National Institute for Health and Care Excellence (NICE) looked at all the data surrounding maternity care and basically said, 'Well, ladies, it looks like over the last 70 years many of you would have preferred to be at home, and it looks like you coulda been there after all! Soz about that.'

Citing the globally respected Cochrane Review evidence, Cathy Warwick, Head of the Royal College of Midwives, announced that having a baby at home or in a midwifery-led birth centre was 'as safe, indeed may be safer, than hospital,' and women report 'higher satisfaction rates and a better birth experience than in hospitals.'

Despite this, only 2 per cent of the UK's 800,000 annual births occur at home. And to understand why, we need a bit of history.

The rise of hospital birthing

The hospitalisation of birth was largely thanks to a general bout of extreme chuffedness at the shiny new NHS hospitals of 1948. The gradual move to get women into labour wards was complete with the publication of the 1970 Peel Report, which stated 'we think that sufficient facilities should be provided to allow for 100 per cent hospital delivery'. It resulted in what Professor Wendy Savage has called 'the biggest unevaluated medical experiment in the world'. As Beverley Beech, who runs the Association for Improvement in Maternity Services (AIMS), says, 'No one asked the women if they wanted to birth in hospital, and no evidence was produced that this would improve care and reduce infant and maternal mortality.'

After 1970, home birth rates fell to an all-time low of less than 1 per cent in the mid-1980s before increasing slightly again to their current levels of 2.3 per cent.

Simultaneously, **caesarean-section** (see page 115) rates rose (now 25–30 per cent in some hospitals despite the World Health Organization saying they should be no more than 10–15 per cent) and, as a result of the 'all that matters is a healthy baby' culture, women are reporting ever greater levels of postnatal depression and post-traumatic stress disorder, with only 50 per cent of women getting the birth they want.

The same Cochrane Review helps shed light on part of the problem, 'The non-familiar environment of a hospital and the interventions may make it less inviting to remain mobile, to actively change between relaxation, joking, intense labour, managing contraction, visiting the loo, bending over a table, shouting at the partner, kissing, going to the kitchen, in short: to remain in control . . . It is easier to lie down on the hospital bed, give up and ask for pain relief.'

How environment affects oxytocin

We now know much more about how and why labour operates, specifically about the role of **oxytocin** (see page 257). This is the 'shy' love hormone that creates contractions and is produced by mammals if they have the right conditions to feel safe, warm, unobserved and calm. Many women feel this way at home but much less so in a hospital room with a swing door, bright lights and unfamiliar faces.

Adrenalin chokes off oxytocin, which is why so many women have yo-yo labours that begin at home, slow down as anxiety rises en route to the hospital ('Who will be with me in labour?', and so on), and then stops completely when they arrive at the ward. Examined and demoralised ('You're only 1cm dilated. Sorry. Go home.'), they return to their warm, cosy, mammalian space and, guess what? Labour kicks in again. This time, once they return to the hospital, feeling like they've been 'getting this all wrong!' they understandably opt for the drugs offered to 'speed things up' and hence begins a series of interventions that make the chance of extra interventions even higher. This is an extremely common scenario for first births and is precisely why so many more women are now requesting home births. It's not whacky. It's not alternative. It's common sense.

Midwives at home births have the experience and skills for positioning a birthing woman (*get off the bed!*) and this rather under-rated thing called 'intuition' that helps them to help the woman help herself (there's a lot of helping in home births).

Pain can be lessened at home

Women who don't fancy a home birth understandably worry about wanting an epidural, but, get this: home birth hurts less. I know, that sounds ridiculous, but it's true. **Fear** causes tension (see page 169), which causes pain, because tension stops your natural pain-killing endorphins from flowing. And as you lie flat on your back in a brightly lit hospital room with your legs akimbo and several strangers coming and going through the swing door, an epidural is, of course, going to feel like your only option. Home birthers commonly use an inflatable pool, a **TENS machine** (see page 314), a spot of **self-hypnosis** (see page 206) and the heavenly delights of **gas and air** (see page 186).

One of the greatest aspects of home birth, however, is the fact that you won't be left alone. On an over-stretched, under-funded maternity ward you might spend a while wondering where the midwife has gone. At the moment, they simply cannot offer the one-to-one care they wish to give (and then there are the inevitable, but distressing, shift changes that leave many frightened labouring women distraught). It's unnatural for women not to know their midwives – all the evidence across the world proves that. But centralised funding systems don't prioritise this basic need – unless you opt for a home birth.

Individual care

You can hire an **independent midwife** (see page 212) or to ask for an NHS home birth even if you have no intention of having one. That way, you will get one-to-one care and be attended at home in early labour but can ask to transfer in when you wish. It's controversial, but it's genius. Why should women be pushed from pillar to post by strangers during their pregnancies because of a one-size-fits-all policy? Men wouldn't accept that. In hospital, you will be attended by one midwife at a time (possibly two for the moment of birth) with obstetricians nearby if needed in an emergency. At an NHS home birth you will have two (or three) midwives with you at all times. In that regard, this is the VIP option.

It's also cheaper for the NHS. A planned home birth costs the NHS £1,066 compared to £1,631 for an obstetric unit birth, £2,369 for a planned c-section and £3,042 for the emergency version. It's cheaper for you too! You save a fortune on not buying snacks from the crappy vending machine because you have your very own fridge (which is normally the biggest plus for dads-to-be) and you don't risk getting a parking ticket.

After the baby is born you can spend the night together in the same bed. There are few times in life when a little privacy is more welcome than when you've just glimpsed heaven (and possibly a little bit of hell), and yet we put women back onto shared post-natal recovery wards, send their partners home and expect them to chat to the stranger in the next bed. And this in an age where we don't even talk on the train!

Problems

'But what if it goes wrong?' Well, sometimes it does. And even NICE advise first-time mums that there is a marginal increase in a poor outcome for home birth (from 4 in 1,000 for hospital birth to 7 in 1,000 for home birth. For second-time mums there is no increased risk whatsoever). It's your own personal choice and your own perception of risk that must ultimately decide if this for you.

Remember that when labour 'goes wrong', it usually happens relatively slowly. Fictionalised TV-births go wrong quickly, because it is the most dramatic scenario imaginable. In real life, a baby's heart rate or a labour itself slowing down happens gradually. And ambulances arrive quickly, hospitals are normally close by and obstetricians are ready and waiting. Midwives qualified to do home births are not idiots. And they won't take unnecessary risks.

We commonly hear the refrain, 'But my baby would have died if we'd been at home.' Sadly, these cases of foetal distress are normally as a result of other interventions that occurred beforehand – these very same procedures simply can't be administered in a home setting. These scare stories are almost never fully understood (even by the women themselves, for whom the idea that there could have been an alternative might be too distressing) and so they circulate, gathering moss and credibility until home birth looks risky.

The most common reason to transfer into hospital from home birth is to access pain relief, particularly for first-time mums who may labour for longer. But these women tend not to regret their choice – they are normally happy to have laboured in the comfortable surroundings of their home until they needed extra help.

Women with complicated pregnancies and underlying medical conditions, which might, for example, affect their ability to stop bleeding after birth, would normally be advised to opt for a hospital birth. If you're getting mixed messages from your care providers about your suitability for a home birth, speak to the consultant midwife. If you aren't getting any joy by working out a solution together, you could also contact the Association of Improvements in Maternity Services (AIMS) whose helpline can advise.

Ultimately, the best place to meet your baby is where you feel safest. That will reduce your adrenalin to a healthy level and allow you to surrender to the extraordinary sensations of giving birth.

For most women that will still be in hospital surrounded by the accoutrements of medicine. But, over time, when your next-door neighbour appears with a newborn on the doorstep and the mum from school is smiling at drop-off having delivered the previous day, it will become normal again.

Pain relief at home

If you're concerned about pain relief at a home birth, here are your options:

- Pool (see page 317)

- Hypnosis (see page 206)

- Massage

- Movement

- TENS Machine (see page 314)

- Diamorphine (ask if your midwife carries this) (see page 138)

Nicola's story

I laboured for 40 hours at home and was therefore seen by three NHS home midwives. They gave us clear options and supported us in every decision we made. I felt truly safe and respected. But on day three of labour, after no sleep and minimal food, we made the incredibly tough decision to transfer into hospital. Our little girl had turned back-to-back and tilted her head. Having dreamt of a natural home birth for so long, I was heartbroken. But I was also tired, tearful and a little fed up. The midwife assured me that I had done incredibly well and that I should be very proud of myself; she even offered to do another four hours at home with me if I wanted. She again gave me clear options and possible outcomes, so I felt confident that I was making the right decision for me and Artemis.

At the Delivery Suite, we were seen by a midwife and doctor who explained our options. I was concerned about the epidural, so they asked the anaesthetist to come and speak to me (bearing in mind that I have never been in hospital in my life and so I had a million-and-one questions). He congratulated me on making it this far, and reassured me that I had nothing to worry about, answering every question with care and compassion.

A few hours later another doctor arrived and I was fully dilated. She informed me that within 30 minutes our Artemis would be born! At this point there was a shift change. The midwives acted very quickly but still managed to explain everything they were doing, what I had to do and where I had to push. True to their word, she was born within half an hour and was straight on boob!

Unfortunately, my womb closed up and my placenta had to

be removed manually. This took just over an hour, but I wasn't aware, as we felt so safe.

After various checks we went home the next day, which I was very pleased about.

We are forever grateful for the safe arrival of Artemis and the excellent care that was taken of us both. We plan to try a home birth for our next baby.

HYPNOBIRTHING/HYPNOTHERAPY/ HYPNOSIS

I would go so far as to say that if you only read one section of this book, read this.

Harnessing the power of your mind is absolutely critical to having a happy birth. It isn't a magic pill that will guarantee you the labour you want. That involves many other contributory factors, not least the position of your baby and the cooperation of your medics. But it is the best side-effect-free-pain-relief technique that can keep you smiling before, during and after your birth. It applies to all births in all settings. Hypnobirthing will teach you so much about your innate capabilities that you will take it with you throughout life. Once there was only the trademarked American brand, 'Hypnobirthing', but now there are hundreds of approaches from thousands of practitioners for your delectation. Each use different 'scripts' and music. They offer different types of training to practitioners and support to clients: either group workshops, online lessons or one-to-one training, as well as downloads to listen to in your own time. But they are almost all fantastic. Ask around for a recommendation in your local area (your midwife is a good place to start) but they all effectively do the same things:

- Give you techniques to stay calm and focused, which you might need when labour kicks in or your caesarean begins.
- Dig out any inhibiting, negative and fearful feelings you might have towards birth from deep within your subconscious mind.
- Help you enter a state of deep relaxation to switch off your busy, conscious brain and let your innate ability to birth your baby take over.
- Give you the ability to turn down painful sensations using visualisations.
- Keep your natural pain-killing endorphins pumping.
- Maximise your ability to generate **oxytocin** (see page 257).
- Distract you from discomfort by taking you to a safe idyll in your mind.
- Give you confidence that your body knows what to do.
- Bring you and your partner closer, because one-to-one sessions with a Hypnobirthing coach can help tease out any issues between you.
- Help you get to know yourself a bit better before becoming a mum.

There are no disadvantages or side effects to developing this valuable skill of self-relaxation. Forget ridiculous stage shows of drunk blokes clucking like a chicken. It will also come in handy at work when you're asked to do a Power Point presentation or when you deliver your Oscar acceptance speech. Staying calm in the eye of the storm is a true life skill. It will also come in particularly handy on maternity leave when your partner walks in with the paper under his arm, sees the half-stacked dishwasher and asks what you've done all day. Thousands of pound's worth of wedding-list crockery has been saved thanks to new mothers being able to breathe deeply.

At The Happy Birth Club, dads are often sceptical until they consider a significant event that they conquered by engaging their minds, such as running a marathon. They accept that having positivity and confidence got them through. A light-bulb moment occurs when they see it as 'mind over matter'.

Of course, women have given birth for millennia without learning the skills of Hypnobirthing. But, arguably, modern life and the medicalisation of pregnancy have helped to erode our birthing instincts. We must work harder now to create external and internal conditions that were readily available to our forebears.

The science?

Think of your brain as an iceberg: the pointy bit, above water, is the part we use every day. That is your conscious mind – your neo-cortex – and it does everything you ask of it. It lifts a spoon to your mouth, it ponders whether lemon in your G&T counts as one of your five-a-day and has you pressing 'search' when secretly trawling ex-boyfriends on Facebook. But everything else is happening beneath the water. All the other drivers that make you do what you do (or do not do) occur beneath the surface: few of us ever truly know what is going on at the back of our minds.

When my third labour wasn't progressing, I had to use a Natal Hypnotherapy download to work out what was blocking my subconscious. I'd spent that pregnancy caring for my newly brain-injured husband, and only by getting into a state of deep relaxation did I recognise that I was more worried about him than me. Hypnosis gave me the key to unlock that barrier.

In labour, the effect of **fear** (whether it's conscious or sub-conscious) on the human body can be extremely powerful (see page 169). When we are scared or threatened, we enter the fight-or-flight state: the blood rushes to our limbs to help us run away. Birth is no time to demonstrate how quickly you can run the 100m; you need as much blood as possible to be directed to the uterus and the placenta to make it function efficiently and to make sure your baby is receiving all the oxygen it needs. Brain scans now demonstrate that if you imagine sniffing a rose, the same part of your brain is activated as if you were actually sniffing that rose. This means that in birth, your mind can't distinguish between a real threat and an imagined one.

Practice is key

Even one Hypnobirthing session is better than nothing, but repeatedly listening to the relaxation and visualisation downloads outside your sessions is key to maximising its benefits. Your body will learn to go into a deeper and deeper trance. It will become easier to slow your pulse down.

By listening to the tracks repeatedly before labour, your body and mind become more familiar with the processes, so increasing your confidence and reducing a lot of the anxiety associated with birth. Then, when you go into labour for real, the suggestions kick in, your body recognises the sensations and thinks: *Oh, yes, we have done this before – this is a trigger for me to relax, stay calm, etc.* The key is to listen to the tracks during the last trimester of pregnancy. The more you practise, the more effective the techniques will be.

Taking time out to lie down and listen to a relaxing download has other helpful benefits: it can help to reduce your daily stress levels, and improve your mood and sense of well-being. Many mums-to-be find it can help them feel energised, closer to their baby and even to sleep better. Aches and pains during pregnancy can also reduce when you take a little time out for yourself in this way.

Some NHS hospitals now offer reduced rate or free Hypnobirthing classes, so ask around.

During the birth

You can listen to the hypnosis scripts as soon as you go into labour. It can be fabulous at keeping you relaxed in the earliest stages of birth while you potter about at home. In order to offset any anxiety that might increase on arriving at hospital, you may want to keep your headphones on. Let your partner do the necessary booking in while you chill – keeping your eyes closed as much as you can (without walking into door frames). Using Hypnobirthing through headphones is a brilliant way to avoid unnecessary conversations you may be expected to have with strangers in hospitals. Genius!

It's vital to remember that if labour is painful, you are not 'doing it wrong'. Personally, I don't believe that there is any way I could have managed a drug-free first birth without Hypnobirthing. It wasn't pain free and in some ways I was wrong-footed by that, as the books had said it would be. But the techniques of breathing and visualisation made the sensations manageable.

It's also worth considering that you may need to give it some welly during the pushing stage. Bearing down with all your might can feel at odds with some modes of Hypnobirthing that promote the idea of staying calm and remaining fairly passive so that your body can do what it innately knows to do. Again, use what you know from hypnosis, but remain open-minded about how you might feel.

It might seem unlikely, but some of the most persuasive stories about hypnosis surround caesareans. Major surgery can be terrifying for some women, so they use the relaxation techniques to enjoy the sensation of lying down and knowing that they will soon meet their baby. Some hypnosis methods offer scripts specifically for caesarean births and there are practitioners who are very skilled in this area.

What will my midwives think?

Many midwives report that they find Hypnobirthing mums fascinating, as they are calmer, quieter and a pleasure to care for. Of course, you will probably still vocalise your feelings! Very few women give birth in absolute silence – regardless of what the tabloids would like us to think about Katie Holmes and Scientology.

The only potential issue for your midwife is that some modes or brands of hypnosis do not permit the use of certain words, as they believe their negative effect on the mind is powerful. So, for example, 'pain' is substituted by 'sensations', and 'contractions' are known as 'surges'. Some midwives feel a bit intimidated or restricted by this in the birth space, but they are increasingly in the minority.

If you know your midwife, you will be able to discuss this with them. If not, include your use of Hypnobirthing on your **birth plan** (see page 71) and any other pointers that you'd like them to know about it.

Shorter labours

Anecdotally, midwives and mothers will tell you that labours using hypnosis are calmer, shorter and less complicated. There have not been enough trials in this area to quote any empirical evidence, or I would. But, frankly, we don't need it. The efficacy of Hypnobirthing is renowned throughout maternity units. Make sure you tell your midwives if you are using hypnosis, as many of the signs of labour do no present; for example, you may not be distressed, you may lie still, gently rocking on a birth ball or floating in a pool, and you may be dilating much faster than it would appear to an outsider. We hear too many stories of hypno-mums being ignored because they didn't seem to be in 'enough pain' to be taken seriously. This is particularly common among those who have had previous births.

I is for . . .

INDEPENDENT MIDWIFE

Survey after survey has established that the one thing pregnant women want is a midwife whom they know. Thankfully, this is now the aim of some NHS hospitals, so ask around – you might be one of the lucky ones.

If not, and a known midwife is important to you, one option is to hire a private, or independent, midwife. For over six months of care and 24/7 availability, they cost between £3,000 and £5,000. There are also other private midwives working in small businesses or social enterprises such as London's Neighbourhood Midwives, who are the first to secure a contract to work via the NHS.

Their job is to care for you clinically, help you towards motherhood and champion your choices – wherever or however you decide to have your baby. There are about 200–250 independent midwives registered in the UK. In recent times, they have faced insurance challenges. Although there hasn't been a single claim of catastrophic outcome against any member of Independent Midwives UK in the last 25 years, they are lumped in with all obstetric outcomes, rendering the premium they must pay as an individual impossible to meet. However, I'm confident that with enough public support, they will survive for generations to come. They are fully trained and are commonly highly experienced. Some work alone; others in groups or pairs.

They may seem expensive, but remember: they care for you throughout your entire pregnancy from the moment you get in touch until – normally – your baby is four to six weeks old. If you consider that a private hospital birth with one overnight stay and no postnatal care can cost as much as £20,000, independent midwives are bloody good value.

Talk to your partner and even wider family, if you believe this is an outlay that would make a difference to you achieving a happy birth. I often find that dads are the driving force behind hiring such support.

This book is all about informing you of your choices, and, frankly, not enough women know about independent midwives – especially first-time mums. They are, however, very popular among second-time mums who wish they had had more continuity of care first time around.

What do you get?

With an independent midwife (IM) you receive more antenatal, labour and postnatal care than you do on the NHS. This will be completely individualised, solely for your benefit and at your convenience. She will monitor maternal health (blood pressure, urine and general well-being) as well as foetal health (heart rate, movement, growth, and so on) at every antenatal appointment. They carry a foetal ultra-sound monitor so that you can hear your baby's heartbeat.

All these appointments will take place in your home, and your midwife will spend time chatting through your fears over cups of tea. Some women like the convenience of an IM coming to their place of work to do the antenatal checks quietly in a side room. The fact is, they are there for you and will accommodate your needs. Normally, they will do home visits in the evenings or at weekends, if that suits you and your partner best. If there are complications that indicate the need for an extra scan or a consultant visit, they will normally come with you at no extra cost.

Once labour begins, the midwife will stay with you no matter how long it takes.

Commonly, their clients have home births, and IMs can be a godsend if you fall into a higher risk category such as **breech** (see page 108), twins or if you wish to have a vaginal birth after a previous **caesarean section** (VBAC – vaginal birth after caesarean), as they are able to take time to assess the whole picture and give you personalised care. But, should you need obstetric care, they will refer you for it and support you throughout. They often know the system and the doctors so well that they help you to optimise both NHS and private resources in your area.

If you do not want a home birth, an IM will offer the same antenatal and postnatal care and will still be at the birth, but they may not be licensed to take a clinical role on the delivery suite or birth centre. Some do – so ask, if this is important to you. Most NHS settings welcome an IM; some may know each other anyway through the small community network of midwives. Even though they are not hands-on in a hospital setting, they can still act as your advocate and help you understand what is happening or what choices you might need to make. At the very least, they ensure you are never left alone. They are also a wonderful resource for your partner who can lean on them if he is worried, or get a breath of fresh air knowing that she is there with you.

Care after the birth

Postnatally, IMs really come into their own. They will tailor their time to your needs, but typically they will come round to you every day in the first week, two to three times in the second week, twice in the third week and once in the fourth week, when they will normally discharge you. They help with feeding and babycare, they will take time to debrief your birth, and make sure you recover and start motherhood feeling great.

You can normally find an IM via recommendations in your area, or go to the website in resources. Meet them: the relationship is the vital ingredient. Don't be afraid to ask if you can speak to someone on the phone whom they have looked after. Explain that you just want some reassurance about whether the process is right for you. The chances are, it will be.

▪ INDUCTION – NATURAL METHODS

The most common day on which women birth across the world is 40 weeks plus 5 days. In France, pregnancy is considered to be 41 weeks. This is because French women have wombs that mature nicely like a fine Camembert while everyone else's goes off like an out-of-date cheese string. So ignore this stupid 40-week deadline. Take the pressure off yourself (like the French do) and stop stressing about your estimated due date (EDD).

If you're 41–42 weeks, however, and desperate to get your baby out, then you can try any or all of these methods. Some are not supported by clinical evidence, but I like them and they have no ill side effects. What have you got to lose?

Eating dates

Jordan University of Science and Technology carried out a study of over 120 pregnant women in 2008 to ascertain whether eating six dates per day for four weeks prior to their estimated date of delivery would affect labour. They found that the date munchers had 'significantly higher mean cervical dilatation upon admission compared with the non-date fruit consumers' (3.52cm vs 2.02cm), and a 'significantly higher proportion of intact membranes (83 per cent vs 60 per cent)'. Amazingly, spontaneous labour occurred in 96 per cent of those who consumed dates, compared with 79 per cent of the non-date consumers. Use of induction drugs was 'significantly lower in women who consumed dates (28 per cent), compared with the non-date fruit consumers (47 per cent)'. And the average latent phase of the first stage of labour was almost half as quick with dates on board (510 minutes vs 906 minutes). The study concluded: 'the consumption of date fruit in the last 4 weeks before labour significantly reduced the need for induction and augmentation of labour'. It's pretty persuasive stuff. So chomp away. It won't do you any harm.

Clary sage

This is a powerful aromatherapy oil that can soften the cervix and might start contractions. Pour some onto a handkerchief and sniff away; however, only start inhaling on or after your EDD.

Some say, even the act of deep inhalation is relaxing, which may explain its efficacy.

Acupuncture

A good acupuncturist with the right experience can make a positive difference – even if it is simply that he encourages you to relax and this drops your adrenalin level.

Raspberry leaf tea

Gulp this down in late pregnancy, because it's good at toning your uterus, and at least one study has demonstrated that it can shorten the second stage of labour and significantly lower the need for a forceps delivery.

Curry

Your bowels lie beside your womb, so the theory is that agitating your guts might trigger contractions. Just a few decades ago, women giving birth in hospitals were routinely given enemas before labour. I'm certainly not advocating that! But a very spicy curry at the end of your pregnancy won't do any harm unless you're also feeling a bit windy, in which case you might want to spend the night in the spare room.

Castor oil

See the same principle above: scatter-bombing the bowl may just get your baby moving, so fed-up mothers-to-be have been necking this candle-flavoured yuck over many generations. If you want to try this, or any similar laxative, have a good night's sleep and start the day with a tablespoon mixed into cereal or fruit juice. Don't stray too far from the loo. A mass evacuation in the supermarket car park is no way to start labour.

Sex

Hahaha! Obviously, heavily pregnant women who can no longer get comfortable without the aid of 16 pillows just love the idea of a good shag. This was clearly thought up by a very clever man who discovered that semen contains prostaglandin, which ripens the cervix. Unless you're betrothed to a sperm whale, your fella probably won't produce enough to make a significant difference. Do not believe reports that it is also effective if taken orally – that's just men wanting blow jobs. Your best bet is to try to have your own orgasm (I know, I know, you may not fancy that either – and if your doctor has advised against it, listen to her). But it does produce oxytocin, the essential hormone for birth, and the pleasurable uterine contractions have been known to kick-start the birth version.

Membrane sweeps

This is classed as 'natural' but it is invasive and would be con-ducted in a hospital before, or as part of, a clinical induction. These will be sold to you as homespun and friendly: no sinister drugs – just a midwife and her finger, and many of us accept them without question. There is no evidence to suggest they work any better than a plate of pineapple (pineapple contains bromelain, which can soften your cervix, but there is little research to support its effectiveness). Most women who have membrane sweeps are due to labour anyway, so who knows if being 'swept' helped? Perhaps their efficacy is psychosomatic: if a woman thinks she will labour due to a procedure, she is more likely to do so; however, a painful and aggressive sweep is not likely to get you into the relaxed state of mind you need to labour. If the sweep is too uncomfortable, you can insist that they stop. Also, a sweep isn't without risk – your midwife might accidentally rupture your membranes, meaning you will be up against the clock to labour spontaneously and thus might face medical induction anyway. Remember, a midwife should still get your permission before she does this. I hear too many stories of women being examined and told afterwards, 'I just did a little sweep on you while I was there.' This is not OK!

Get a late scan

Based on the fact that your brain and body are connected and you're more likely to labour if you're not anxious, a late reassurance scan might be just what you need to put your mind at rest. London's top two teaching hospitals, King's College and UCL, now offer scans as routine at every 40-week appointment, and it helps to determine each individual's course of action – which may, in fact, be to do absolutely nothing. A sonographer can check the amount of water around the baby, its position and the efficiency of the cord and the placenta. These are the main worries with an 'overdue' pregnancy. This knowledge can be very empowering when you're negotiating your need – or lack of it – for induction.

Reflexology

Thousands of women testify to the fact that this brought on labour, so if you think it's worth a go, seek out an experienced reflexologist with specific experience. Make the most of the time out in their chair and relax, breathe deeply and think positively about the excitement of meeting your baby soon.

Hypnobirthing

It could be that there is an emotional, mental block holding you back from labour. See Hypnobirthing (page 206) for an explanation of why this may work.

■ INDUCTION – MEDICAL

Before we talk about inducing labour, let's look at the numbers:

- In the UK, a baby is considered term (fully cooked) at between 37 and 42 weeks.
- A post-dates pregnancy is over 40 weeks.
- A post-term or prolonged pregnancy is beyond term: 42 plus weeks.

A quarter of all UK births are induced, and this number has consistently risen over the last ten years. Doesn't that strike you as odd? What's going on here: a lack of patience on the part of doctors and mothers-to-be? An eagerness to control nature even if it might not be in the mother's or baby's best interests? Is evolution causing us to gestate for longer? Who knows? The very fact that women are 'diarised' a confidence-dashing induction date at their standard 40-week antenatal appointment could be a contributing factor too.

Some women are having inductions that are 100 per cent necessary, due to them or their baby suffering a medical condition such as obstetric cholestasis, diabetes or high blood pressure; however, more women than ever are starting labour through induction drugs simply because they are 'overdue' and are told that this increases the risk of the baby being adversely affected. 'Risk' is a concept that has been completely mucked up by modern maternity services, litigation and inadequate assessment methods. If we had a system of individualised care, many fewer women would be categorised as high risk; however, women are so damn good at protecting their young before they're even born, we're sensitively tuned to conversations about risk and due dates.

Of course, risk is a very personal concept, and each woman will view risk as an individual: would you cycle with or without a helmet or take an illegal drug? Perhaps you wouldn't risk telling your best mate her hairstyle makes her look like a child in the 1970s? Everything we do in life involves risk. So, when considering whether to do X or Y, there is no risk-free option. All you can do is choose the option with the risks that feel right for you. Take a deep breath if you're faced with the induction dilemma, and know that you can still have a happy birth and consider all of this.

Your **obstetrician** (see page 249) has a legal obligation to give you all the information you require before agreeing to an induction. Induction to meet an overdue baby is not right or wrong if the choice is made by a woman who has an understanding of all the options and associated risks. And there are few decisions more difficult in pregnancy than working out if you want to be induced.

The changing lengths of 'normal' gestation

Very few women experience a prolonged pregnancy anymore, mainly because most hospitals have an induction policy at 41 weeks. But if one in four British babies is now being induced, we have to question whether this protocol is right? Are we really to conclude that Mother Nature has got herself all confused about gestational timing when she got it right for so many years before?

It's worth factoring in that genetic differences might influence what is a 'normal' gestation time for you. A 2011 study found a familial link that must be considered: if your mother, grandmother and even dad/granddad were the result of long pregnancies, it seems you may offer the same go-slow route to your baby. Interestingly, a 2016 study of 500 women concluded that those in the third trimester 'taking individual zinc, folic acid or iron supplements in combination with a multivitamin were twice as likely to birth beyond 41 completed weeks than those who did not'. I'm not suggesting that you stop taking your daily vitamins. This clearly needs greater investigation. But, these researchers concluded, 'Well women consuming third trimester individual micronutrient supplements in addition to multivitamins experienced a longer gestation at term, increasing their risk for postdates induction of labour.' With our diets getting better, longer pregnancies might be something the medical world has to get used to.

But my doctor says that if I go overdue I'm placing my child at risk!

In theory, after 42 weeks the placenta starts to shut down. But there is no actual evidence to support this either. Dr Harold Fox, writing in the respected, peer-reviewed journal *Archives of Disease in Childhood, Neonatal Edition*, states: 'There is, in fact, no logical reason for believing that the placenta, which is a foetal organ, should age while the other foetal organs do not'. Midwives report seeing signs of placental shut down at 37 weeks and also, big juicy healthy placentas at 43 weeks. A scan might help to put your mind at rest if you want reassurance.

You may also hear that your baby will grow huge and the skull will calcify, making moulding – when the baby's skull bones adjust – and therefore birth, more difficult. Again there is no evidence to support this theory, and babies are pretty good at finding their way out of their mother's expandable pelvis.

Top marks to those of you who spotted the contradiction: if the placenta stops functioning, how does the baby continue to grow so well?

The serious concerns

The real concern with waiting beyond 41 weeks is the increased chance of the baby dying before it is born. That's some seriously big shit to consider. There is literally no sane woman on this planet who could shrug off a suggested induction when told that her baby might die. But there is much scaremongering around this sensitive subject. A Cochrane review, which objectively summarised all the quantitative research examining induction versus waiting, concluded 'There were fewer baby deaths when a labour induction policy was implemented after 41 weeks or later.' That's pretty convincing; however, it went on to say: 'such deaths were rare with either policy . . . the absolute risk is extremely small. Women should be appropriately counselled on both the relative and absolute risks.' No matter how considerate and time-rich your obstetrician is, we'd bet few pregnant women hear 'risk of death' and digest the difference between the 'relative' versus 'absolute' risks of waiting versus induction.

Let's boil this down: if you are induced at 41 weeks, your baby is less likely to die during, or soon after, birth than if you did nothing. That feels very categorical. But, the chance of your baby dying is tiny either way – less than 1 per cent. That's 30 out of every 10,000 for those who wait or 3 in 10,000 for those induced. Therefore, 1,476 women would be induced to prevent 1 stillbirth at 41 weeks. That's 1,476 labours being unnecessarily (and painfully) medically induced. But after 42 weeks, the risk does increase significantly with a stillbirth rate of 1 in 1,000 (according to R.L. Dekker, 'Labour induction for late-term or post-term pregnancy' in *Women Birth*, August 2016).

Nevertheless, reviews are only as good as the research they review, and there are some concerns about the quality of the available research. The World Health Organization recommends induction after 41 weeks based on Dekker's review but acknowledges the evidence is 'low-quality evidence. Weak recommendation'. Another review of the literature in the *Journal of Perinatal Medicine* concluded: 'It is not possible to give a specific gestational age at which an otherwise uncomplicated pregnancy should be induced.'

Part of the problem with this unsatisfying data is that is focuses on *what* is happening rather than *why*; for example, congenital abnormalities of the baby and placenta are associated with longer pregnancies and this may account for the increased risk of death rather than the length of gestation. Quantitative research also takes a general view rather than assessing the risk for an individual woman in a particular situation: does this woman come from a family of women who have a longer gestation timeframe?

It's vital that more research is conducted into the implications of induction for women who go overdue, and it's important that the currently known risks are discussed as part of the information a woman uses to decide what is best for her.

What happens now?

If you have exhausted all **natural induction** methods (see page 215) and decide that you are informed and happy to commence an induction, your doctor will explain all the steps to you.

There are three basic steps to induction. You may find that you can avoid some of these steps, but prepare to face all of them, and be happily surprised if you don't need to. If your waters have broken naturally, the term 'augmentation' rather than 'induction' is used to describe getting labour started. This is because it is assumed that your body has started the labour process itself.

On a very basic level, it may be useful to ask yourself:

- Am I simply too fed up with being pregnant to continue? How much happier would I be if my baby was now out?
- Starting birth medically creates further risks that require further monitoring. Am I happy with that?
- Are the risks involved in continuing the pregnancy greater than the risks involved in induction?
- Induction goes only one way: to birth. Am I ready to take that journey, as there is no going back?
- Use the **BRAINS** (see page 279) questions in all your medical discussions and seek second opinions if you have any doubts.

Induction – the procedure

During pregnancy the cervix is closed and firm, keeping your baby, placenta and amniotic fluid safely enclosed. The cervix can still be closed even if you are having contractions. To chivvy the cervix along, some practitioners offer a membrane sweep during pregnancy – even before you have hit your EDD (see page 162). In doing the sweep, they are trying to separate the membranes of the amniotic sac from the lower uterus to release prostaglandins; however, there is little evidence that this is effective and a Cochrane Review concluded, 'Routine use of sweeping of membranes from 38 weeks of pregnancy onwards does not seem to produce clinically important benefits.' They go on to say that it 'needs to be balanced against women's discomfort and other adverse effects'. So you may wish to try a sweep to get your sleepy baby moving, or you can say, 'No thanks, my vagina ain't no chimney and it doesn't need sweeping.'

If you don't mind a vaginal examination, however, it gives the midwife a chance to assess the condition of your cervix. If it's already soft and sufficiently open enough to break your waters, this will be step one. A long metal hook (amnihook) will gently pop your sac of waters through the neck of the womb. This should be largely painless, but you will still benefit from relaxing, breathing deeply and softening your muscles as much as you can. If this is successful, induced contractions should be more effective, as your baby's head will press harder on the cervix with no water to cushion the sensation. This alone may trigger efficient contractions meaning that you avoid further interventions. Of course, there are other risks associated with artificially breaking waters, so from that moment your care providers will be clock-watching. The more examined you are, the greater your risk of infection.

If your cervix is too firm and closed, making breaking your waters impossible, artificial prostaglandins will be applied to the cervix as a gel or pessary. Your baby's heart rate will then be monitored by a cardiotocograph (CTG), as these drugs can cause hyperstimulation of the uterus, causing foetal distress. You may also feel 'prostin pains', which are sharp, strong pains sometimes accompanied by contractions.

You may need two attempts with re-insertion of prostaglandins. Ideally, you would be given the first dose at night and allowed to go to bed in the hospital. This can take hours or days because you must wait about six hours before re-assessment and re-insertion. This may be enough to sway you into labour, and you would therefore skip the following steps; however, you are still having an induced labour and will usually be treated as high risk.

Once your cervix is primed for contractions and no amniotic fluid is in the way, all that's needed are contractions. In a natural spontaneous labour, **oxytocin** (see page 257) is released and helps the uterus to contract regularly; thereby altering your mindset to produce natural, pain-killing endorphins. In an induced labour, artificial oxytocin (Syntocinon) is given via a cannula on the back of your hand directly into the bloodstream. It only works on the uterus to regulate contractions and is so powerful that it can send your uterus into over-drive – hence your baby will be monitored closely using a CTG.

Strong contractions
It's anecdotally recognised that artificially stimulated contractions are more painful than natural contractions. The physiology of the contraction might be the same, but during an induced labour the rhythm of contractions and their intensity increases more quickly than most natural labours. Women are not able to slowly get acclimatised to the sensations or use natural endorphins to temper their perception of pain. In modern parlance, they tend to 'climb the walls'. The circumstances and environment that normally surround an induction are obviously clinical in nature, meaning that women must work harder to maintain their self-belief and stay relaxed. Inductions are more likely to result in the use of an epidural. Artificial oxytocin will also be used to deliver the placenta.

Inductions can be a very good way of avoiding a caesarean section. But a prolonged and difficult induction can be more challenging for a woman than a calmly planned caesarean section.

Stacey's story

After preparing for weeks using natal hypnotherapy with a view that I wanted as natural a birth as possible, the news that I was to be induced due to developing gestational diabetes was not welcome. My husband and I convinced the specialists to allow me to reach my due date, and as it grew closer we did everything to encourage our baby to arrive: acupuncture and reflexology, but to no avail. I do, however, believe that they prepared my body for a smoother labour. The day arrived and the drugs themselves were easily administered. We escaped and went for lunch. But the drugs accelerated my early labour and we eventually returned to hospital for monitoring. The next few hours were probably a bit worse than if I had gone into labour naturally; however, when the time came, I still managed to walk to the ward and the staff, I think, were even more sympathetic towards women who had been induced! I eventually succumbed to stronger painkillers, as I understood that being induced means operating within slightly different parameters. I just needed to accept that. Our baby arrived at 7am in the morning, less than 24 hours after my induction and earlier than they had originally intended to assess me! Our little girl arrived safely into the world with no complications. Yes – being induced meant that I couldn't have the natural labour I wanted, and it did mean I ceded an element of control that I wanted to maintain; however, it did mean that my baby arrived safely and that I was looked after in the process (and if you like to plan, the element of knowing when your baby will arrive is quite useful). There is definitely nothing to be afraid of.

INTERNAL EXAMINATIONS

Internal or vaginal examinations are when a midwife sticks her fingers up your tinkle and measures (using her skill – not a ruler) the dilatation of your cervix. Think carefully about whether you want one. Will it change your course of action? You won't need to do anything to speed up your contractions if your labour is progressing normally, so is there a benefit to knowing if you're 2, 4 or 8cm dilated?

If you arrive at hospital and a midwife reveals that you are 'only 2cm' will you feel demoralised? Getting to 2cm is actually no mean feat, but it might feel disappointing if it's delivered to you in such a fashion. Partners can step in here to lift your spirits and keep you positive, but you may be happy to ride out the sensations, not knowing how dilated you are and see what happens next. If you have a home birth with a known midwife, the chances are you will never have an internal exam at all.

Please remember that although they might be presented as inevitable, internal examinations *are entirely optional*. It is useful for hospital staff to know how dilated you are, as it can give them a vague idea of how long your labour may have to go, and they are planning which beds, midwives or rooms they will need over the next 24 hours. But that's not your problem. If you do not feel like an exam, you can politely refuse.

Some midwives are very experienced and can use other cues without the need for an internal examination, but they may still be under time pressure, which makes such exams unavoidable. Discuss their approach to internal examinations in your antenatal meetings.

Typically, it can be dads who want to know how dilated their partners are. Sometimes (sexism alert) men aren't good at operating within a very fluid time frame. Plus, in their defence, they may have the car on a meter and don't want a ticket. But making a labouring woman feel rushed is never, ever a good idea. Talk about this with him before you're in labour.

If you do want an examination to see how well established your labour is (if, for example, you want an epidural and are considering if it's the right time), try to relax, breathe deeply, call on any **Hypnobirthing** skills (see page 206) and know that it only takes a moment. It shouldn't be painful, but it might be uncomfortable.

K is for . . .

K – VITAMIN

Vitamin K is offered to all new babies in order to prevent something called haemorrhagic (wow – spelled that right first time!) disease in the newborn. Haemorrhagic disease can occur at any time in the first 12 weeks, and vitamin K completely protects babies against it.

About 1 in 10,000 babies are deficient in vitamin K, which

is a clotting agent in healthy blood and therefore leads to an increased risk of bruising and bleeding. This is no laughing matter – such bleeds can cause serious conditions including death. Unfortunately, unless there is a strong history of bleeding disorders in the family, there is little way to know which babies are susceptible. Premature infants are at greater risk as are those who have difficult instrumental deliveries. So, in order to mitigate any risk, the majority of babies across the world are routinely given vitamin K in two forms:

1. By injection within the first 24 hours of birth.
2. By oral drops given soon after birth; at 7 days old and at 4 weeks (if baby has been given formula milk during this period, they do not need the extra drops).

Amazingly, until the late 1980s, babies were given the injection without parental consent – mums would simply see a bruise and a plaster on their baby's thigh and ask who did this. Now, midwives must get verbal permission from one or both parents. If you don't want your child to have the vitamin by injection, you will probably be visited on the ward by a paediatrician who may attempt to diplomatically twist your arm. But you still have a choice. Most hospitals will have oral drops on their midwife's prescribing guidelines, and your community midwife will administer the drops needed on days seven and 28. Or, you may be shown how to administer them yourself. Or, if you are only given two doses (as can be the case with some hospitals) you will need to go to your GP to get a prescription for the last dose. There really are no specific pros and cons. It's basically whether you want your new baby to have an injection or not – your choice.

You can put your requirements on your **birth plan** (see page 71).

L is for ...

LABOUR

It's no coincidence that birth is termed 'labour', because it is often hard work – especially first labours. It might be useful to think of it as two types of effort: one that happens naturally, internally, without you having to even think about it, as your uterus is so clever. And the type that involves real physical and mental endeavour – pushing, breathing, squatting, believing in yourself and, possibly, mooing like a cow. Every labour is different: there isn't one linear route that all births follow. The duration, the intensity and the effort required will be different for everyone. And the ways in which women 'manage' their births are wildly different.

Firstly – and this might seem an odd place to start – but what would you say is your 'personality type?' This is likely to affect how you feel about labour and the sort of environment that would suit you. Women who are inclined to be 'in control' need to work harder to switch off and trust those around them; they may also like using external distractions such as apps to time contractions, or pain relief such as a **TENS machine** (see page 314) that they control. If you are an anxious type, get empowered with **Hypnobirthing** skills (see page 206) and consider having a **doula** (see page 150) by your side. Someone who is easily intimidated might need to equip her partner with the knowledge to act as her advocate.

Or you might prefer to go with the flow, switching off the busy, neo-cortex part of your brain, closing your eyes and introducing external coping strategies as and when you feel you need them.

Remember: it's all about *you*, because you are doing something amazing.

But regardless of your characteristics, physically we're all pretty much the same when it comes to labour.

Labour is measured in stages: first (cervix dilated to 10cm), second (pushing and birth) and third (delivering placenta). As a labouring woman, it doesn't matter if you can pass a test on such facts. For millennia women didn't know this detail. They simply hunkered down and birthed their young. But your birth attendants might use these phrases, so keep them on your mental list.

Perhaps, more helpful is knowing that labour pain is normal and is helping your baby to arrive safely. For many women, having a baby is an intense experience, which can be unnecessarily frightening if you don't understand what's happening.

Early or latent labour

For first babies, early labour – that is the time spent dilating to roughly 3–4cm, can be long and unpredictable. It may last any time between, on average, 5 and 20 hours. For others (especially second-time mums), it progresses smoothly after a few hours into active or established labour, during which you progress to full dilation. It depends on many factors, including the position of your baby, how relaxed you are and the strength of your contractions. You can call your midwife/place of birth at any time, once you think labour has begun.

The first signs of labour

You may feel:

- Intermittent tightening of your tummy or back.
- Period-like pains.
- Excitement and adrenalin – rushing to the loo to empty your bowels.
- Your waters may break.
- You might have a 'show' (see below).

If you experience any of these, inform your midwife by phone. They will want to talk to you – not your partner – and will probably keep you chatting while they assess your condition down the line. Basically, they want to see if you can carry on talking through a contraction. If so, they will probably suggest you give it a few more hours and then call them back.

Your uterus, or womb, is a massive muscle that is carrying your baby, placenta and a couple of litres of water. It's a strong, water-tight, perfectly sized bag, and such a sturdy construction means that it needs to work hard to open up.

Contractions gradually soften, shorten and open up the neck of the uterus – the **cervix** (see page 133). Throughout your pregnancy it has been closed and plugged with mucus to keep out infection (I know, 'mucus plug' is a terrible word combination, so let's move swiftly on). Now the cervix needs to 'ripen' and open, so that your baby can be born when it is fully dilated to about 10cm in diameter.

As a result of these changes, the mucus plug (sorry) might come out. This is called a 'show', but it wouldn't pack out a house in the West End. It looks a bit like white or pink jelly and can be stained with blood. You might find it in your pants or down the loo. Or you may not have one at all. If this is your first baby, your labour might start within hours or days of the show.

Try to be patient during early labour. This is a marathon, not a sprint. Eat, drink, stay at home, potter about and keep yourself distracted.

Waters breaking

This is often a good indication that your baby is ready to arrive.

If your waters do break at this point, they may do so in one gush that will leave you in no doubt that they've broken (or 'gone'). It's not exactly like the movies, where customers white-water raft down the supermarket aisle, but you might notice a surprising warmth and realise that people are throwing bread at you, as you're surrounded by ducks. There is actually only about 2 litres of fluid at full term, and it's unlikely to all come out in one go. You won't need your swimming goggles. What most women don't realise is that your body will then carry on producing more amniotic fluid and keeping your baby well. You'll need to wear maternity pads to soak up the moisture and save your sofa. Alternatively, your waters might trickle in a way that makes you wonder if you've simply peed your pants.

Pay attention to the colour of your **amniotic fluid** (page 32). It should be straw-coloured or possibly a little pink, if it has absorbed blood from the show. If your waters clearly contain blood, tell your midwives immediately. Similarly, brown or green waters might indicate meconium (baby poo) and may signpost a different route to birth than you had planned (but not necessarily, so don't panic).

Once your waters have broken, your medical support will probably want you to go into labour within 24–72 hours. This is a big difference, and you should check on your particular carer's protocol. There is a risk that your baby could develop an infection, hence the anxiety around letting women go beyond that time limit. See **augmentation of labour** (page 55) for advice on what to do in this instance.

Contractions

These are simply the horizontal and vertical muscles of your uterus contracting and relaxing to release your baby. Like any muscle use, this can have an accompanying discomfort. Try to think of it as sports pain, rather than illness!

You'll have your own rhythm and pace of labour. As a rough guide, early contractions are usually more than five minutes apart, and only about 30 seconds or 40 seconds long. In between them you will feel completely normal – if a little anxious.

There are lots of coping strategies that you and your partner can use at this stage:

- Sleep
- Listen to your body – move around until you feel relatively comfortable
- **Tens machine** (see page 314)
- Sit on a well-inflated Swiss ball
- Massage
- Listen to your **Hypnobirthing** downloads (see page 206)
- Think positively!
- Relax and go to a 'happy place' in your mind's eye
- Homeopathy
- Aromatherapy
- Eat and drink as your appetite demands
- Balance movement with rest and sleep
- Have a wee at least every two hours
- Have a warm shower or bath

Stay at home for as long as possible unless you have been advised not to due to medical complications. It is much better to arrive at your place of birth in established labour – you will be seen more quickly and are more likely to get what you want, be that the use of a birthing pool (see **water birth**, page 317) or an **epidural** (see page 155).

See **contractions** (page 135) for more detail.

Active or established labour

In active labour, the frequency, length and intensity of contractions become increased. If you are having your baby at home, you will probably want your midwife with you for reassurance. If you like stats, during active labour, your cervix opens from 3 or 4cm to becoming fully dilated at 10cm.

Contractions are more powerful but will usually start gradually, building up to a peak of intensity, before fading away again. This is why it can be useful to think of them as waves. You probably won't be able to talk through these contractions. You may have to stop and breathe, or moan through them. Keep your jaw loose and let any noises flow out. Women often make extraordinary noises in labour – that's normal. Contractions may come as often as every three to four minutes, and last between 60 and 90 seconds, giving you less time to rest between them. But between contractions you will be able to talk, move, kiss your partner and prepare yourself for the next one.

As your labour becomes stronger, you'll probably lose your appetite, feel or be sick (your body cleverly clearing your digestive system so that all resources are focused on your baby's arrival). You may feel like walking around and being mobile. You may wish to get into the pool. This can be wonderful. But try not to get in too soon, as it can slow contractions down. Ask your midwife's advice.

Contractions in this active phase tend to maintain their momentum and open your cervix more rapidly, but it may still be many hours before your cervix is fully dilated. Take it one step at a time, and remember that each contraction is bringing you closer to meeting your baby.

You may be offered **gas and air** (entonox – see page 186) to take the edge off the contractions. This can be fabulous. But, keep in mind that if you're aiming for a natural birth without an **epidural** or **diamorphine** (see page 138), you might want to wait until you really need the entonox – ideally in the pushing stage. If not, go for it. It will keep you relaxed before an epidural arrives.

You might be offered **internal examinations** (see page 229) throughout your labour. Remember that they are optional and probably best avoided unless knowledge of your dilation is to be used to change your plans or time pain relief.

Transition in labour

This happens at about 8–9cm dilation and tells your birth attendant that you're doing brilliantly and will soon be ready to push. This is just like in a triathlon: during transition you change one mode of transport to another – and in labour you may literally want to get on a bike and leave the hospital. In transition, women go a bit loopy and decide that they're going home. Don't be freaked out – you're not going insane. This is the time when you might feel utterly demoralised and say you can't do it and your husband is never coming near you again. You will insult the midwife, criticise the décor and announce that you have always hated your mother-in-law. In transition you will think everything you read in this book is utter bollocks.

You may have less frequent, but much stronger and longer-lasting, contractions. Sometimes they come in double waves. Each one may peak, start to fade, but then increase in intensity again, before fading away completely.

It's common for waters to break just before, or during, transition. As your cervix becomes fully dilated, you may have another small show of blood. Having support and reassurance will help you to get through this stage. Thankfully, there can be a lull at the end of transition, when the contractions pause. Don't panic. Some midwives call this the 'rest and be thankful' stage. Some women even take a little nap! This is nature's way of letting you and the baby rest before the pushing stage. I know – amazing isn't it?

Pushing

In movies, women are told when to push and everyone stands around the bed shouting *'push!!'* as though she is approaching an Olympic finish line. This is nuts. There is no evidence that cheerleading positively affects birth.

If you haven't had an epidural and you're upright, comfortable, safe and relaxed, pushing will probably feel completely instinctive. It's not something that you can fight against or ignore. It's a bit like the sensation of vomiting – but in a downward motion. The uncontrollable wave that makes you throw up is very similar to the pressure you feel when needing to bear down and push your baby out.

It may be useful to think of this more as 'breathing your baby out' rather than pushing with all your might until your eyes go red and your brain pops out of your ears. Use your breath: exhale slowly with each downward sensation and inhale deeply as the contraction fades. This will keep you and your baby well oxygenated.

Don't be afraid if it feels like your baby is coming down and then popping back up again. This is good. It means that your body is stretching slowly and cleverly rather than quickly. Go off to the happy place in your head, allow your body to open up, listen to music and try to be patient. You're doing the most amazing thing in the world and will soon have a beautiful baby in your arms.

Some contractions will feel expulsive, as the baby moves down. Some will feel more stretchy as the tissue inside the birth canal makes way for your little cherub. Listen to the midwife's/obstetrician's suggestions as the baby gets closer. They may ask you to pant with shallow breaths, rather than push, once the baby 'crowns' – that is, the head is almost ready to be delivered. This is to protect your **perineum** (see page 272) and to ensure that this last stage is as comfortable as possible. It can be irritating to be directed in this way, but a skilled birth practitioner knows what they are doing and should be listened to.

Some hospitals will have guidelines about the length of time they will 'let' you push, but it is roughly about two hours. I don't like the word 'let' – some women can push for three hours without any damage being caused to their pelvic floor. But it's impossible to know whom – so discuss this with your practitioners beforehand and make an informed choice. Ask them to explain their protocol, then, if you agree, you can feel reassured. But make it clear that you would like to try more upright positions if pushing is taking too long before opting for an assisted delivery.

If you have an epidural or an assisted delivery by ventouse or forceps, you will work with your obstetrician to get your bubba out.

Breathe long, deeply and rhythmically, listening to their guidance on timing your pushes.

Crowning

This is the moment when the top of the baby's head is out and will soon be born. For most women (particularly with their first baby), it stings. The female body is incredibly stretchy and can do remarkable things that you can't yet imagine – but we know this is the moment that most women fear. It can be hard to stay relaxed and not fight the sensation. Keep your shoulders down and your jaw slack. Women who don't have an epidural often report that gas and air comes in handy for this latter stage.

Once the head is delivered, don't panic. That's the hardest bit done. If you're in water, this can feel scary, but remember your baby has just come out of water and is still getting oxygen through his cord. There is no rush. Sometimes, contractions can stop for a few moments at this stage. It may only take one or two more pushes to deliver the baby's squishy, lovely, snuggly body and then you will have created and birthed a brand new human.

Well done you!

Skin to skin

As long as your baby is A-OK and doesn't need any extra help (the vast majority of babies are OK, remember), he should be placed directly in your arms and onto your chest. It can be lovely to pick up your own baby, but be mindful of the length of the cord – adrenalin and enthusiasm are in abundance, and you don't want to tear the cord or pull at the placenta. The benefits of skin-to-skin contact with mum immediately after birth are numerous, including the regulation of the baby's temperature; the benefits to their microbiome and simply because it's just totally awesome to see your baby for the first time. The chances are, you'll be overwhelmed with how amazing they are. But don't be too shocked or disappointed if you don't feel that immediate rush of love. There is a tendency to over-sentimentalise this moment. It can blow your mind as blue tits begin tweeting overhead and a harp starts to play – or it can feel more like, thank-god-that's-over-now-get-me-a-cuppa-and-I-can-check-out-this-little-guy-in-good-time. Again, everybody is different.

Delivery of placenta and cord clamping

Your work isn't quite done yet. If you want a 'physiological' or 'natural' third stage, you will deliver the placenta naturally without any drugs. This is only an option if you have had no other drugs except **gas and air**. It can take between 5 minutes and 1 hour, but it's a boneless, squidgy organ that will emerge without much effort. You won't notice much discomfort, as you'll still be marvelling at your son or daughter. The very size of the placenta might freak you out a bit, as they are normally about 22cm in diameter and 2cm thick. The midwife should never pull on the cord to force the placenta to break away, as this can cause huge problems for mum, including haemorrhaging. They will check that all the placenta has been removed and take it away for disposal.

If you wish – or have had other drugs during labour – you will have a painless injection (Syntometrine) into your thigh, which forces the placenta to come away safely. This is called 'active management', a 'medical third stage' or a 'controlled cord traction'. It is always used in the event of a placenta that isn't coming away as quickly as the midwife would like. Syntometrine has negligible side effects, which can include nausea, sickness and headache. It can also raise blood pressure.

The midwife will then clamp and cut the cord (see **cord clamping** – page 137) to stop the drug reaching your baby.

Write on your **birth plan** (see page 71) which option you would prefer if all has gone well.

M is for ...

▪ MICROBIOME

This refers to the bacteria that live on and in our bodies. Scientists believe that they have only scratched the surface in learning how it affects our physical and mental health. But they are certain that it is 'seeded', or switched on, during birth. When babies are born vaginally, they absorb vital bacteria that live in the birth canal. Typically, they have a much more diverse microbiome than those born via **caesarean** (see page 115). Those who study the microbiome believe that a lack of bacterial diversity might impact a child's future health. There is some speculation that this is why babies born via c-section are five times more likely to have significant allergies and asthma. But don't despair if you have a c-section. A second, crucial phase of seeding your baby's microbiome occurs when they are placed on the breast soon after birth. This can obviously be done at most c-sections. If this isn't possible – for example, if your baby is moved to special care – you can hand-express breast milk into a tiny syringe with the help of your midwife.

As with all options, read up and decide for yourself. There is a fantastic documentary, *Microbirth*, which examines the entire phenomenon and is certainly worth a watch.

▪ MIDWIFE (LABOUR WARD)

In the UK, we are fortunate to still have a maternity service staffed predominantly by midwives: caring, qualified, sensitive women (and men!) whose job is to support, advise and empower pregnant women to birth their babies. But our birth rate has increased faster than the number of midwives who are qualifying, leaving a shortage of almost 3,000 of these guardian angels. Hopefully, you will meet only kind and compassionate midwives with the time to care. Having a midwife that you know has been proven to reduce mother-and-baby mortality, increase breast-feeding rates and lower the use of pain relief. So why not do your research and try to find a hospital that can offer this service? They are on the increase.

MORO REFLEX

This is worth knowing so that you aren't scared witless if you see your baby's arms shaking. It's named after the chap who spotted it – Austrian paediatrician, Ernst Moro. Within all healthy, newborns is a reflex that scientists think is a hangover from our primitive past hanging about in trees. If a baby feels that it is falling, it will fling its arms and legs outwards and draw them back up quickly – appearing to shake quiet violently. If you place your baby quite quickly on the changing mat for example, you might see this happen, and it can really freak you out. The reflex isn't doing your baby any harm, and if they do cry they can normally be settled quite easily with a reassuring cuddle. The Moro reflex will normally disappear by three to four months of age. It's one of the standard means of assessment at a newborn baby check, as it's a good indicator of the health of the central nervous system.

Some babies are more shaky than others and can demonstrate a Moro reflex even in their sleep. Sometimes, this is so intense that it wakes them up. You know that feeling when you're having a dream and you feel that you're falling and you wake with a start? It seems to be like that for babies. It's quite cute to witness in a sort of funny-but-I-really-shouldn't-laugh way – so to help your nervous little cherub, try swaddling and carrying baby in a sling.

MOVEMENT

Feeling your baby's first movements is a lovely, bizarre, mind-blowing moment. You won't believe the kicking, tumble-turning and general merriment going on inside you. Most women will feel movement between 16 and 24 weeks.

Your baby will have its own natural pattern of movement. After 24 weeks the movement will increase until 32 weeks and then it will stay roughly the same until birth. It is not true that babies move less towards the end of pregnancy. They should carry on moving up to and during labour.

Reduction in movement can be an early warning sign that your baby is unwell. Don't wait until the next day if you are worried that their movements have slowed down or stopped completely. Almost half of women who had a stillbirth noticed their baby's movements had slowed down or stopped.

Be aware of your baby's daily patterns: do they wriggle more at night or in the day? On a busy day, you may be unsure about whether you have felt movement. Lie on your left side, relax and concentrate on their movements for no longer than an hour. If you are still concerned, do not delay in getting checked out. A deviation from your normal pattern should always be checked out.

Have a cold drink or sugary snack to see if this wakes the baby up.

If your baby's movement has reduced, you might turn to a hand-held monitor, phone app or Doppler to check your baby's heartbeat. But even if you do detect a heartbeat, it doesn't mean your baby is well if it's not moving.

Trust your instincts. You know your baby better than anyone, so be insistent if you feel something is not right. You are the mother and you know best. If you are at all concerned, make sure you get checked and, if necessary, ask for a second or even a third opinion.

N is for ...

NON-INVASIVE PRE-NATAL TEST (NIPT)

This is a blood test that can be taken from a mother in early pregnancy to predict some types of genetic foetal abnormality. It comes under various brand names, but it is most commonly known as the Harmony test. It might not be routinely available on the NHS in your area, but do ask. If you wish to access the test privately, it will cost about £500 including two scans and a blood test.

Taken at 10 weeks or later, the test is predictive to more than 99 per cent in Down's syndrome, 97.4 per cent for Edwards' syndrome and 93.8 per cent for Patau's syndrome. This hugely reduces the need for invasive testing by chorionic villus sampling (CVS – see **genetic testing** page 188) or amniocentesis and the miscarriage risk that they carry. An ultrasound scan is performed just before the blood test to date the pregnancy and to check that the mother is not carrying twins or more. If you have used an egg donor, ask your obstetrician whether the Harmony test would be of value to you.

If you are able and prepared to pay privately, anyone who wants extra reassurance about the normality of the pregnancy can have the test. Older women (particularly over 35 years) and those who have already had a chromosomally abnormal pregnancy are more likely to opt for the test. It is helpful for those who have had a previous sex chromosome abnormality such as Turner's syndrome. It can also tell you the sex of the baby by 10 weeks.

The procedure

It is a very simple procedure. The mother has to sign a consent form and one for data release. After the ultrasound scan a blood test is taken from the vein in the arm. There is no risk from having the test. Two tubes need to be fully filled and they are sent away for analysis. Privately, the result is usually available within 10–14 days. It takes a little longer on the NHS.

There is a 1 in 30 chance that no DNA is obtained. This is not a positive or negative test: it is an unsuccessful test. A private clinic will usually offer a repeat test free of charge. This is usually successful.

The result is expressed as a probability. It is a screening test and not a diagnostic test. A good test result gives a risk of a chromosomal problem of less than 1 in 10,000. A bad result gives a risk of greater than 99 per cent. A high-risk result would then require an amniocentesis or CVS depending on the clinical situation. You would be sensitively counselled about this.

Depending on how many weeks pregnant you are, you would still have the opportunity to have a 12-week **nuchal scan** (see page 248) privately or within the NHS. The focus of the 12-week scan would change as you would already have the result of the Down's syndrome test. The 12-week scan would thus look at the baby in detail for structural (physical) abnormalities. Remember, these may exist without a chromosomal abnormality. You will still have the opportunity to have the later scans, such as the 20-week scan, as before. If the Harmony test is negative, it is important that the person conducting the 12-week scan is aware of this.

There may still be structural abnormalities such as spina bifida, heart defects and a poorly growing baby that will only be seen on scans and often not until later, so these scans should still be undertaken.

NUCHAL TRANSLUCENCY SCAN

For the last ten years, doctors have been using the results of the nuchal translucency scan to advise pregnant women and their partners on their risk of having a baby with Down's syndrome or other abnormalities. The nuchal translucency scan looks at the skin fold on the back of the baby's neck at about 12 weeks. This has been further refined by looking at the nasal cartilage of the baby using an additional blood test to identify two pregnancy hormones. This is the combined test and has achieved a predictive value of about 82 per cent. Women with a high risk have an option to proceed to chorionic villus sampling (CVS – see **genetic testing** page 188) or amniocentesis. These are invasive tests that carry a miscarriage risk of about 1 in 100. If you have an abnormal nuchal scan, ask about availability of **NIPT** (sometimes called the Harmony test – see page 246), as this will soon be offered on the NHS and can help clarify the likelihood of your baby carrying abnormalities.

O is for ...

OBSTETRICIAN

Hopefully, you will never have to see an obstetrician during your pregnancy and labour. Women without complications receive midwifery care on the NHS, and many studies have demonstrated that this is safer for mum and baby; however, you may prefer to be looked after by an obstetrician and be willing to pay for this private option. But, be prepared to ask questions of your doctor in order to establish that they are right for you and will provide the sort of time and attention that you deserve and expect. At The Happy Birth Club I have drawn upon the brilliant wisdom and experience of Professor Donald Gibb of The Birth Company in Harley Street.

Professor Gibb on the role of the obstetrician

Donald's sessions with our parents-to-be are firm favourites, and his calm, reassuring manner must be a natural drug of its own in labour. His woman-centred approach to birth makes him the perfect person to offer an insight into the role of the obstetrician and his thoughts on birth:

What is the difference between a midwife and an obstetrician?

A midwife looks after women having a straightforward pregnancy and birth, which most women have.

Obstetricians in some countries (USA, Australia, continental European countries, usually with a private model of care) also do this; however, obstetricians have a wider remit than midwives in looking after women with high-risk pregnancies. These might be pregnancies complicated by medical disorders such as diabetes or heart disease, and so on. They also look after women with other reproductive issues such as previous miscarriage, previous caesarean section and complications of birth. The relationship between midwives and obstetricians is important to facilitate the involvement of the doctor at the right time when complications develop.

What questions should you ask when looking for a private obstetrician?

Is he or she available when you are due to give birth? If not what are the cover arrangements with another doctor? What is their experience of pregnancies like your own? What type of birth do they feel comfortable with (see 3 below.)? What are the contact arrangements during pregnancy, and particularly around the time of birth? Does the obstetrician give you a mobile phone number? You must also ask yourself after you have met him or her: do you like them? Consider the As, are they: affable, approachable, able, available, affordable?

What are the potential pitfalls of hiring a private obs?

Make sure that they are clear about their availability. This is not just when they might be on holiday or away at a meeting. What is their local availability? What are their NHS commitments that might detain them at a critical time?

Make sure they are in tune with your expectations. It is convenient and easy for a private obstetrician to do a planned caesarean section or induction of labour. It may not be so convenient to spend all night in the delivery suite for a first birth. Beware that most obstetricians are not enthusiastic about water birth.

Under what circumstances is an obstetrician a necessity?

If you have a complicated pregnancy or have had a previous caesarean section, or if you require a repeat caesarean section, it is best to have an obstetrician. In the face of life-threatening complications (rare but possible) it is essential to have an obstetrician.

OP (OCCIPUT POSTERIOR)

A baby that is OP is in the occiput posterior position. This means that although she is head down (rather than **breech** – see page 108) the back of her skull (the occipital bone) is in the back (or posterior) of your pelvis. You may also hear this position referred to as 'face up'. Many more babies are posterior at the beginning of labour than when they're born, due to the natural rotation that occurs on descent. It is estimated that as many as half of all babies are OP when labour starts, with only 4–10 per cent of babies remaining so at birth. But the percentage of babies who are OP at birth is higher among first-time mothers.

Babies during labour (without an epidural on board) do a lot of rotating, as the contractions push them downwards so that their position changes several times until shortly before birth. For this reason an OP presentation should not be a cause for panic or alarm.

In order to avoid your baby slipping into an OP position, try not to slouch on the sofa in a U-shape. We all do it, but it creates a sort of internal hammock that can encourage baby's back to slide round. Instead, lie on your side on the sofa and sit upright in chairs. Better still, sit on a Swiss ball or on a reversed chair and lean forward over the back of it. You may not want to spend hours watching TV like that, but being mindful of your posture can help prevent your baby turning OP. There are two fantastic websites with advice for optimising your baby's position (see Resources).

OSTEOPATHY

Osteopathy can be a godsend for pregnant women who develop aches, pains, niggles and more serious musculo-skeletal concerns. That's why I brought Lisa Opie (MBEm Most, BSc hons) into The Happy Birth Club. She is a brilliant osteopath who teaches the couples about self-care during pregnancy and beyond. These are her words of wisdom.

Lisa Opie on osteopathy

During pregnancy, you will see significant physical changes happening to your body, and the inevitable weight increase can put a considerable strain on your musculo-skeletal system. Your posture is constantly changing throughout the three trimesters, as seen in the illustrations opposite. Expectant mums can put on as much as 10kg (1½ stone) of weight once we account for

How posture changes in pregnancy

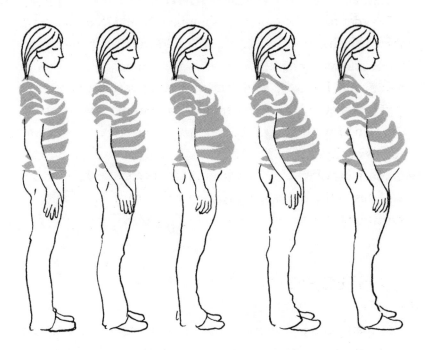

the baby, water and the placenta. This weight increase, combined with the hormone relaxin, puts enormous stress on joints, organs, ligaments and other tissues of the body. Relaxin prepares the pelvic floor, or pelvic ring, for birth. It allows the ligaments around the pelvis to relax – which is great; however, it also affects all ligaments throughout the body during and for some time after pregnancy. It makes you more flexible, which might sound promising, but ligaments are responsible for stabilising our joints, therefore lax ligaments can mean lax joints, so stretching and yoga should be modified.

Osteopaths are trained to treat pregnant women and understand the natural changes that take place and how

Facet joint

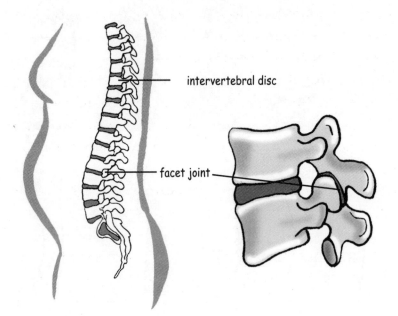

intervertebral disc

facet joint

the body adapts. They understand the fears and emotions that go with pregnancy and having a first child. They will generally avoid or heavily modify their treatment in the most vulnerable weeks 12 and 16.

Common complaints that can be treated with osteopathy

Low back pain This is generally due to the increase in lordosis, or arch of the low back, as the stomach size and weight increases. This shortens the low back muscles and puts strain on the small weight-bearing joints of our spine: the facet joints (see above).

How to manage low back pain:

- Stretch your low back with knee hugs. This may get more difficult further into your pregnancy as your stomach grows, so seated knee hugs one at a time might be more comfortable.
- Stretching and keeping your upper, middle back and ribs mobile will also reduce the load and stress in your low back. A good way to do this is sitting on a Swiss ball keeping your hips facing forwards and rotating your upper body.
- Standing rotations holding a Swiss ball or a pole are also a good way of mobilising your ribcage.

Gluteal or buttock pain Buttock pain (or piriformis syndrome), is common during pregnancy.

How to manage gluteal or buttock pain:

- Modify the seated single-leg knee hug (described above) by angling the knee towards the opposite shoulder. It's a good way to stretch your buttock muscles.

Hip flexors and hamstrings Due to the increased arch in the low back, the hip flexors and front-of-thigh muscles can become short and tight. This, in turn, will pull the low back into more of a lordosis and overstretch the hamstrings.

How to manage hip flexors and hamstrings:

Try the following to stretch all three muscles (the stretches should be strong but not painful – if your muscle is shaking, ease off):

- Kneeling hip flexor stretch: Kneel on a soft mat or folded towel on your right knee (or the side that requires stretching). Make sure that your left knee is directly over your ankle and your left hip is at a 90-degree angle. Engage your core or lift your pelvic floor, if possible. Tilt your pelvis backwards by tucking your 'tail' under and squeezing your glutes. To gain a stronger stretch, push your left hip/knee forward slightly and lean back. Hold for up to 20 seconds and repeat, if necessary, on the other side.
- Standing quadriceps or front-of-thigh stretch: Stand on your right leg, holding on to a stable surface if necessary. Bend your left knee, grab just above your ankle and pull your thigh back so it is level with your right thigh. You will feel the stretch down the front of your thigh. Keep your torso upright and try not to lean forward. Tilt your pelvis under by tucking your 'tail' under to gain a stronger stretch. Hold for 20 seconds then swap sides.
- Standing hamstring stretch on step: Using a chair or wall for support, raise your right leg and place the heel on the step. Keeping your knee straight, lean forward from the waist, looking forward and keeping your back straight. You should feel a stretch down the back of your thigh. Hold for 20 seconds and then swap sides.

There are many classes that are designed especially for pregnancy, including Pilates, yoga, aqua and even personal training in the gym. All these are good ways to stay mobile and reduce the risk of pregnancy-related musculo-skeletal problems. It is important to remember, however, not to embark on any strenuous exercise regime if you didn't do anything before your pregnancy.

OXYTOCIN

This is the most important hormone you will need during labour (and sex). It flows with abandon when you feel safe, happy, warm, cosy and emotionally liberated. If you are a finely tuned Formula One car about to glide magnificently towards the chequered flag of motherhood, oxytocin is the grade-A fuel to power your engine.

Hospitals offer a synthetic version of it in a drip for **inductions** (see page 215) or to **augment** (see page 55) or speed up labour, but the natural version is way more effective. (Think bog-standard petrol from the pump compared to Ferrari-grade, hand-filtered, uncontaminated compounds of pure magic.)

Oxytocin is also known as the 'shy hormone', because it will not come out to play if it feels observed and under threat. Create a dark, safe, warm space and it will tentatively emerge, but it is sensitive and can easily disappear once again if these conditions are interrupted by bright lights, a perceived threat (by, say, a vaginal exam that you really don't want) or a change of midwifery shift.

The enemy of oxytocin is adrenalin, and we can thank Mother Nature for the clever relationship between the two. This symbiosis is the reason we evolved. As mammals, it's not in our interests to labour if we feel scared: our young would have been eaten by sabre-toothed tigers long ago.

This is why so many women experience yo-yo labours. Picture this: they are at home, cosy, eating a mint Aero under a blanket and watching *Tattoo Fixers* when labour starts. But they're informed and know not to panic. They chill, do nothing, stay calm. They go to bed. Then they wake up at 2am and decide things are cracking on, and they waddle into the car with a sleepy partner. On the drive, they start to worry: have I packed everything? Where will we park? Who will I see? What if I don't like my midwife? Is my hubby going to be OK? What if the pool isn't available? What if this reeeaaallllyy hurts?.

They arrive in the brightly lit hospital where they hear someone vocalising their birth and by now (unless they're aware of the importance of oxytocin and using all my tricks to maintain **calmness** – see page 132) they are poised for action; their fight-or-flight mechanisms are firing on all cylinders. The blood is rushing from their uterus (where it's needed most) to the legs in order to run away from the perceived danger.

This is when labour commonly stops. Kaput. No contractions. They're shown into triage, where they're examined behind a curtain and told that they're 'only 1cm'. They feel silly. They were sure it was happening! They're sent home, as it's a busy ward and there's nowhere to wait.

Back home, disheartened at the false start, they climb back into the cosy, dark warmth of their own bed; they finally breathe deeply and their shoulders drop – then they wake up an hour later with strong contractions. This time, they go in, shaken by the false start, but in some discomfort. Yet again, contractions slow down in the unfamiliar environment. Now they are convinced that they're 'doing it all wrong' and a midwife finds them quietly crying in the reception area. After another dispiriting examination and the pain that comes from feeling so tense, the midwife starts to feel for her and says kindly, 'Come on, let's get you on a Synto drip to get things going.' They mean well. But this poor lady is 'failing to progress' and from that point onwards, hooked up to a drip and a monitor (and probably on her back on the bed) the birth is under clinical management and thus the chances of extra interventions increase. Most importantly, she is not happy.

This pattern is the reason more second- than first-time mums have home births. But fear not, simply being aware of this scenario empowers you to avoid it. You can still choose a hospital birth and keep your happy hormones flowing. See Partners (page 262) and Calmness (page 132).

P is for ...

PAIN

At one of the early sessions on The Happy Birth Club course we do a word-association exercise to gauge how our participants are feeling about labour. The answers to the question: 'Give me one word that you associate with labour' are usually variations on the following:

Pain
Ouch
Agony
Magical
Scary
Terrifying

Sadly, very few women view birth as little more than impending physical torture. Perhaps this is because we have a very simple relationship with pain: if something hurts, it must be bad, and medicine can make it stop. (Those drug companies have pulled an absolute blinder in brainwashing us into this view.) But pain isn't always bad, and we need to reframe our thoughts on the concept of pain in relation to childbirth.

Bad pain from illness or injury is never nice. And in those instances, be thankful that we live in a land where doctors can administer drugs to ease our symptoms.

But pregnancy is not an illness. Birth is not comparable to any other physical event, and yet it tends to hurt. So, against this backdrop, it's a big ask to view the physical sensations as 'good'.

Even without venturing into *Fifty Shades of Grey* territory, there are many types of pain that are doing us 'good': teething – the act of growing teeth, which, I'm sure you agree, are extremely useful; the pain that comes as a result of strengthening your muscles after exercise; and growing pains – a side effect of developing your limbs. Labour pain falls into this category. It's great pain for the very best reason: getting your baby out into the world. Labour pain shouldn't be feared. Every tightening is simply your uterine muscles easing your baby into the world.

If you still aren't convinced, I can assure you that labour is not agonising non-stop for the duration of your labour.

How much actual pain might you experience?

The average first stage of labour lasts between 12 and 18 hours, so a woman in a 15-hour labour might 'enjoy' 3 hours of one contraction every 15 minutes, lasting around 20 seconds. That's only a total of 4 minutes of discomfort for the first three hours.

Then you may be looking at another 3 hours contracting every 10 minutes for 30 seconds. So that's another 9 minutes of ouchy.

That's only 13 minutes of pain in the first 6 hours.

Between contractions you will feel as normal as you do right now, reading this: utterly pain free; in fact, you might even feel elated and a bit high, as the cocktail of endorphins and hormones combine to take the edge of physical discomfort.

Throughout the next 3 hours, contractions might come in waves every 5 minutes lasting 45 seconds, equalling 27 minutes of contractions.

Now you only have 6 hours left. Three lots of 60-second contractions in every 10 minutes means that you've only got to manage another 108 minutes of intermittent discomfort until you meet your baby. And the whole 60 seconds is not agonising – the pain ramps up as the contraction intensifies to a peak, but quickly eases off again.

You've been in labour for 15 hours, or 900 minutes, and you've only been in 'pain' for 148 of those minutes. That's only 16.5 per cent of your labour in which you will need to breathe deeply, visualise your happy place and remember that you are a lioness. The other 83.5 per cent of the time you felt absolutely normal – in fact, you probably felt blooming marvellous.

All I can really say is: don't worry about pain. I promise you – women who have difficult or traumatic births never talk about the pain. They say, 'Nobody listened to me', 'I didn't know what was happening' and 'I felt dehumanised.'

The important thing to think about is who you want with you at the birth to make you feel at your most relaxed. Think about where you would feel happiest and whether you are fully prepared: mentally, physically and practically. Nobody will give you a trophy for bypassing the drugs. It's not a competition – do what makes you happy. But without drugs, labour is usually more straightforward with a quicker recovery and fewer long-term problems. Pain is temporary. A baby is forever.

▪ PARTNERS

As you approach your due date, you are likely to start thinking about the role your partner can play during your labour.

Obviously, not all partners are 'dads-to-be'. One of my all-time favourite birth stories involves a lesbian couple who nobody on the labour ward had identified as such, until the baby was born and 'dad' took off 'his' shirt for skin-to-skin contact. The doctor's expression, when faced with not one but two pairs of boobs, was apparently a picture of sheer befuddlement. All of the advice here applies to same-sex couples too, so please forgive the momentary emphasis on male partners.

When it was more common for women to have babies at home, men were generally found down the pub during labour. Birth was women's business.

In the 1970s, with fewer women-centred home births, greater sexual equality and more male obstetricians, dads began to be invited into the labour ward. It quickly became the norm for dads to be present during labour. This isn't to say that it suited all dads-to-be, or their partners, and we're too quick to assume that this is the way it has to be.

When considering the role your partner can play in your labour, it's critical that your partner is allowed to choose whether or not they wish to be there. You may feel disappointed if they don't – but, trust me, an anxious, squeamish or terrified dad-to-be can be a worse birth partner than no dad at all.

World-famous obstetrician Michel Odent, who pioneered **water births** (see page 317) and campaigned for men to be present at labour, has revised his thoughts on the issue after 35 years catching babies. He now believes that men should not be at labours, because women spend too much time worrying about whether their partner is OK and that can affect their own levels of tension, compromising the production of oxytocin.

If your partner is feeling nervous about being present at the birth, talk honestly and openly about whether an alternative birth partner would be better for you both. That might be a mother, sister, mother-in-law, **doula** (see page 150) or known midwife. Whatever you choose, it's paramount that you have this conversation sooner rather than later; however, a calm, loving, strong, supportive partner whose neck you can smell and hands you can hold can be an absolute gift in labour. They are your 'guardians of **oxytocin**' – the hormone women need to labour effectively (see page 257).

Remember, a hospital-based birth environment with its unfamiliar rules and regulations can make birth partners edgy, nervous and totally unsure about what to do or whom to speak to. But most partners really want to help – be it by stroking your back or politely asking for an epidural.

It's important to discuss your hopes, fears and expectations with your partner. Contrary to the romanticised idea of pregnancy, it's common for couples to have their most blazing rows during these 40 tense weeks. Don't feel bad if you've considered walking out of the front door and never coming back. There has never been so much pressure on you as individuals and as a couple. The responsibility of a baby's arrival can feel utterly overwhelming – not to mention the hurdle of labour to get over. But there is lots you can do to ease the stress.

Try this

Whether your partner is keen to be present at the birth or not, here is an exercise that you might like to do together:

1. Pick a moment when there are no time pressures, and switch off your phones!
2. Without looking at each other's words, you and your partner should each make a list under the following headings:

   - Practical
   - Physical
   - Emotional

3. Yours should be a list of things you would like your partner to do in labour. Your partner lists what they feel they would be able to do.
4. You should also write down three things your partner definitely should not do. (Imagine the room in which you're having your baby, and picture anything that they might say or do to seriously piss you off.)
5. Compare and contrast your completed lists, and try not to have a massive row. The chances are, you will end up laughing! This exercise will encourage empathy from both of you. It will also help manage your expectations before birth. It will help both of you become clearer about the way you will work together in labour; for example, do you think your partner would function better with specific tasks to focus on? Many men are solution focused, so consider giving him a specific 'job'. Just telling him to be 'supportive' is probably too vague!

The three lists below will give you ideas about the types of things your partner could do. All these suggestions are relevant whatever type of birth you have: natural, epidural or abdominal (**caesarean**, see page 115), and most can apply to any birth partner (mother, sister, doula, and so on), but some are quite obviously for the person you have sex with (you'll see what I mean).

This section is written *for* your birth partner. It won't take long to read and contains everything they need to know.

Practical

1. **Travel** Be in charge of directions. Have a glove box full of coins. Some hospitals don't take cards at pay and display, so work out your options (or, better still, visit) the place of birth and get your head around the parking.

2. **Food and drink** The uterus is a big muscle that will be working out for hours. Imagine going to the gym for two days and not eating! (See **birth bag** – page 65 – for what to take.) Your partner may not want to eat anything at all (or even if she does, she may throw it up anyway) but little mouthfuls will keep her energy up.

3. **Pillows** You are in charge of taking two pillows in distinctive pillow cases (not white, see page 67). Being comfortable in early labour is really important (and you may even be allowed to borrow one to nap in the chair if she lets you).

4. **Music** Take charge of the iPod/CDs – whatever she fancies to get her through the upcoming endurance event: whale music or Eminen? Whatever makes her feel invincible or calm.

5. **Lights** Make the room feel as homely as possible. Dim the lights (and dim them again once the doctor has left the room and left them on full).

6. **If she wants to be up** and about, feel free to move the bed against the wall (if there is one) and make sure there are mats and balls that she can use to get comfy and keep moving.

7. Between you, use your **BRAINS** (see page 279). Remember, birthing women need time and patience. That doesn't always fit within a hospital's scheduling. Your mum-to-be is more important than a hospital timetable.

8. **Take photos** but discuss beforehand what type she would like – distant and moody or close-ups of her most precious parts. Charge the camera or phone battery and take discreet shots when she is looking at her best.

9. Read the **birth plan** (see page 71). Several times.

10. **Watch for people coming into the room** who do not introduce themselves. Smile and hold out your hand, 'Hello, I'm ... this is my wife ...' If they *still* do not tell you their name, ask for it. At least 20 per cent of birth practitioners do not volunteer their names. They may enter a room and look at the monitor or straight at your wife's vagina. When else does that happen in real life? It's not acceptable. Take charge of it.

11. **Most midwives and doctors** are lovely and attentive. Some are not. If you really do not like the manner, tone or attitude of your medical support, the chances are you aren't the first person to have thought this. Kindly, but assertively, ask the midwife on reception when your midwife came on her shift. If she has half an hour left, go with it. If she is on for the next ten hours, you can politely ask for an alternative. If you are met with resistance, ask for the supervisor of midwives to be bleeped. One will be on duty 24/7 and can sort out any problems. Use her to make sure you have a positive experience. You do not need to struggle through with someone who makes you feel angry or vulnerable. You can do this outside the room so as not to stress out your partner.

Physical

1. **Be a leaning post** Human beings make great birthing posts. Let your magnificent woman relax her arms around

your neck and lean into your chest. Do not fall over. Gravity is a girl's best friend in labour.

2. **Shoulder press** Gently press her shoulders down. Women will often try to lift away from the pain of contractions, and tension causes shoulders to lift and necks to stiffen. Gently easing them down will remind her to relax and get back into her body.

3. **Try pressing quite firmly** into her lower back with every contraction – many women find this helps with the pain. But if she doesn't like it, stop.

4. **If you have done some Hypnobirthing** (see page 206), you can quietly say some of the phrases from the downloads to keep her calm and grounded.

5. **Stay away from her** Use your instincts. If she starts to pace and move around like a wild animal, give her some space. Sit calmly in the chair and tell her you are there when she needs you.

6. **Hold her head** If your partner is in the birth pool, you might want to hold her head as she floats on her back. Stroke her hair out of her face and tell her she is wonderful.

7. **Remind her** to go for a wee if she hasn't been for some time (the midwife should do this, but they sometimes forget).

8. **Distract her** Throughout labour, but especially in the early stages, it is great if you can keep your lady distracted from the business going on inside her. Chat about noncontroversial issues (this isn't the time to discuss the mortgage or suggest an open relationship).

9. **Be funny!** Laughter is a great way of producing **oxytocin** (see page 257) and relaxing the cervix. She fell in love with your jokes – this is your big moment. Just don't take the piss out of how horrific she looks right now.

10. **If labour is stalling,** ask for 30 minutes of privacy. Oxytocin is produced by hugging and kissing. If you can, lie on the bed and chill out. Nipple tweaking and clitoral stimulation are brilliant ways of getting labour moving – obviously she doesn't need you for that.

11. **If she has an epidural,** stand in front so that she can rest her head on your chest. Gently stroke her arms, tell her she is amazing and that you're so excited to meet your baby. Even if you are shitting yourself, don't let her know. She will absorb your anxiety.

Emotional

1. **Your partner is the most important person** in the room. Sorry, but it doesn't matter if you are hungry or tired. Keep it to yourself, say you are going to buy a drink (and ask does she *and* the midwife want anything?) then go and get a breath of fresh air, a sandwich and a strong coffee. It's OK for you to take a break if you need one.

2. **Women in labour** are almost always scared. You can help make her feel safe. Be completely present in the room – *do not* look at your phone unless she wants you to text the grandparents and has specifically asked you to do so. Do not look bored (even if you are). Women never need to be more grown up than the day they birth their babies. The same goes for you.

3. **Protect her** Hospitals are busy places in which birth practitioners don't always have time to consider privacy. Stand at the door if she is frustrated at people popping their heads around the door. *Smile,* introduce yourself, ask if you can help and say that your wife just wants some quiet time.

4. **Be emotionally strong** for your partner – remember, she loves you and you're going to be a great dad. Then when your baby is out, you can blub like a total Jessie.

PELVIC FLOOR

Even if you never want to go trampolining with your children, the pelvic floor is vital to every woman's health and well-being. Pregnancy and labour put it under considerable pressure and strain. This can have long- and short-term consequences for you physically, sexually and emotionally. Life can be miserable if you are having to wear incontinence pads as a matter of course.

Some women find that they may leak a little for several days or weeks after birth. Do your pelvic-floor exercises before birth as often as possible. You can start doing them again the day after you give birth.

Incontinence is not a normal effect of labour, and talking openly about such issues has really helped to remove the stigma and improve awareness.

If you do find that your continence is badly affected by pregnancy and labour, speak to an expert and consider your options. The best place to start is your GP. If your problem is sufficiently bad, surgery might be required at a later date. If you intend to have more children, you are probably best advised to wait until you've been through all the births you want beforehand.

I brought Hannah Cooksey onto our team, as I hated the idea of women feeling unable to live full and happy lives after birth because their pelvic floor was letting them down. She is a physiotherapist with expertise in women's pelvic health. Here is her insight and knowledge:

Woman's anatomy

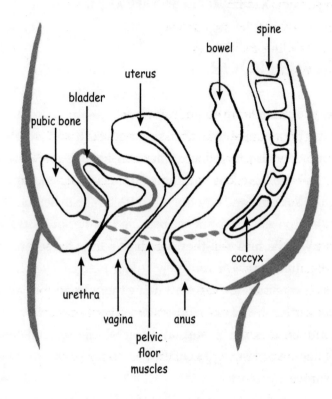

Hannah Cooksey on pelvic floor exercises

What is the function of the pelvic floor? It supports the
bladder, uterus and bowel, and assists normal bladder
and bowel function, preventing leakage (incontinence).
Sexual fulfilment and the ability to orgasm might be
compromised if the pelvic floor loses its tone.

The pelvic floor becomes weakened by:

Pregnancy
Childbirth

Chronic cough

Being overweight

Being generally unfit

Changes due to the menopause

Long-standing constipation

Heavy lifting

How to strengthen your pelvic floor

You can do a number of exercises to activate and strengthen your pelvic floor. Aim to do 30 short and 30 long squeezes each day in groups of 10 using any of the suggestions below:

- Pull in the muscles you use to try to stop yourself passing water/wind.
- Pull your back passage towards your belly button.
- Pull your sitting bones together without squeezing your buttocks.
- Imagine picking a pea off the seat using your vagina.

Always be careful to avoid the following:

- Bearing or pushing down.
- Holding your breath; instead, try to pull in your pelvic floor while you are breathing out.
- Squeezing your buttock muscles.
- Bracing with your abdominal muscle.

The pelvic tilt – lower back stretch – to relieve lower back pain

The exercises can be done in a variety of postures, but

generally try to imagine that you are trying to pull your tailbone in between your legs or that you are tucking in your bottom.

A nice position to try is leaning on a counter or the back of a chair with your elbows or with your hands resting on a box (see opposite). Now try to pull your tailbone between your legs. You should feel a stretch in your lower back – make sure you are not just bending your knees. Hold for 5–10 seconds and repeat 10 times.

The cat stretch
To do the cat stretch (see opposite), start on your hands and knees, aligning your wrists underneath your shoulders, and your knees underneath your hips, with the spine in a neutral position. Keep the neck long, then tip the pelvis forward, tucking in your tailbone until your spine naturally rounds. Now, pull your navel towards your spine and drop your head. Hold for 5–10 seconds with each movement, using your breath. Repeat ten times.

PERINEUM

This is the posh name for the bit of skin and muscle between your baby hole and your bum hole. In birth, you will be amazed at how mahoosive your lady cave can stretch. The question is, what can you do to minimise any damage to this precious area. There are gadgets for sale that claim to help minimise your risk of vaginal tearing or need for an episiotomy. The science behind such products is decidedly flaky. Nevertheless, some women find that knowing their tinkle can stretch as wide as a tennis ball prior to birth is an eye-opener that gives them confidence in Mother Nature.

Lower back exercises

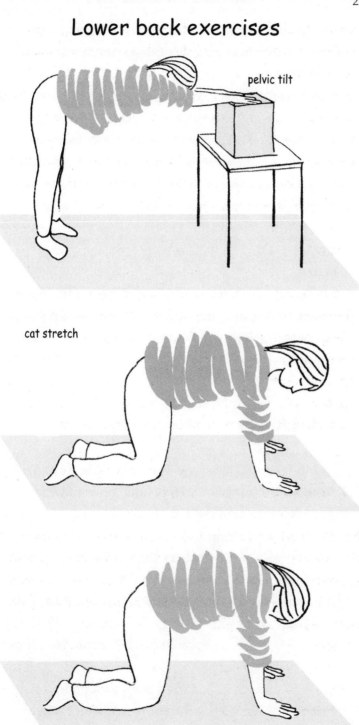

pelvic tilt

cat stretch

Of course, few things are as scary as having your ninky-nonk torn asunder, and there are other things you can do to help protect your perineum.

Perineal massage involves using a special perineum massage oil (such as Weleda, see Resources), finding a bit of privacy and washing your hands. Then insert your thumb into your special place. Exert gentle pressure in a downward, half-circular motion towards your back passage (a bit like when you clean out a mug with a sponge – stay with me here) so that the perineum is stretched a little downwards. Do this a few times a week for a few minutes at a time. It will keep the area supple in preparation for labour.

Other factors in preventing tears are adopting effective, upright positions during labour, an absence of induction drugs, a skilled midwife and the ability to mentally relax your lower regions when it's the last thing you want to do.

POSITIONS

You may find that you instinctively move your body into comfortable positions during labour. Hopefully, your midwife will also encourage you to remain upright, active and involved in positions that are good for getting your baby to move downwards and then smoothly out into the world. On the following pages you'll find some positions that you might try. (Obviously the swimsuit is optional – but how else could I demonstrate these without an x-rated certificate?!)

Positions to try in early labour

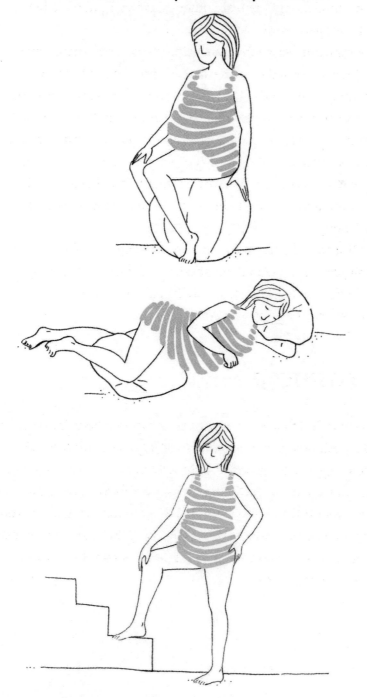

Positions that may feel comfortable in established labour

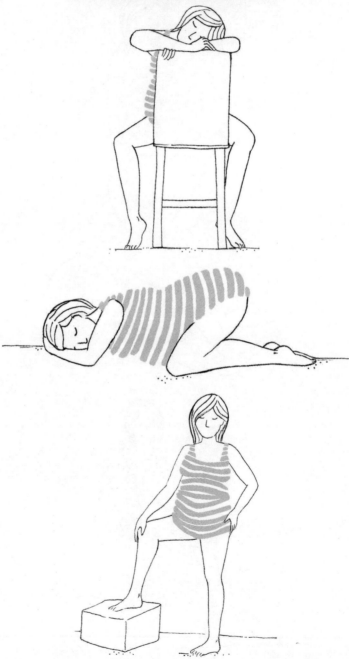

Positions for pushing

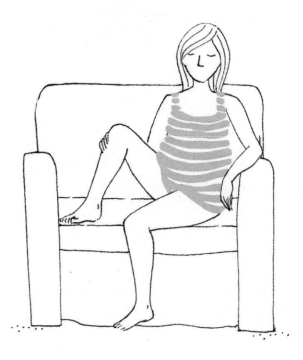

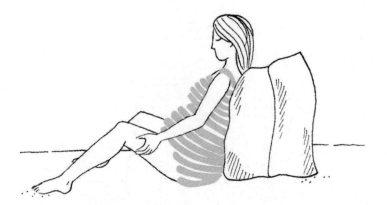

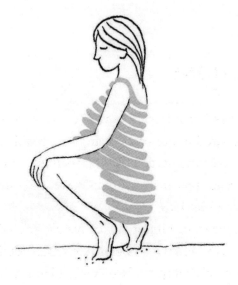

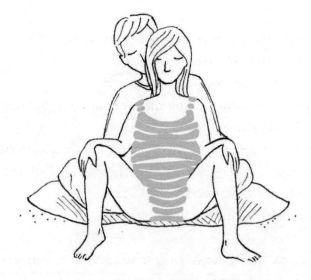

Q is for ...

QUESTIONS

There is no need to assume that your doctors are wrong, but you must be prepared to question them. The trouble is, being faced with white coats and name badges is incredibly intimidating; it's easy to become forgetful and submissive. I recommend this clever little acronym: BRAINS.

It can be used in pre-labour conversations with your birth practitioners, in labour to navigate different options, and you can even remember it when faced with dilemmas about feeding, sleeping or immunisations with your new baby. I even use this in life when faced with difficult decisions regarding work, kids and, even, relationships. The principles apply to almost everything.

Ask yourself or your medical practitioner:

B – what are the *benefits* of this to me/my baby?
R – what are the *risks* to me/my baby?
A – what are my *alternatives*?
I – what is my *instinct* telling me? And ask the doc what their instinct is telling them.
N – what will happen if we do *nothing*? (for example, in labour, if you feel rushed by hospital protocol, requesting half an hour to see what happens is sometimes all you need).
S – ask all these questions with a *smile*!

Some say that the S is for shout or scream! And there may be times when you need to assert your demands quite forcefully – but in hospital, as in life, you will probably get a better outcome if you talk to folk with politeness and a well-intentioned smile.

R is for ...

REIKI

Aches, pains and niggles that we would normally fix with a quick painkiller and a glass of water, challenge us to find alternative therapies in pregnancy. Try not to view this as a hassle but an opportunity. Women who use **acupuncture** (see page 23), **hypnotherapy** (see page 206) or even reiki often discover that they develop a habit for life. Olivia Southey is our **Hypnobirthing** coach and **doula** (see page 150), who increasingly practises reiki and sees extremely positive results. This is her expert insight.

Olivia Southey on reiki

What is reiki? Reiki is a gentle therapy in which the therapist transmits energy through the laying on of hands. You remain completely clothed during the treatment and it isn't a massage, but the therapist places their hands gently on you in a sequence. You may feel lovely warm, glowing sensations, or tingly feelings, or you may sense colours or sounds during treatment. The premise behind reiki is that everything is made of energy and that we all have a kind of life force within us that keeps us healthy and happy if it flows around the body smoothly and there is plenty of it. But when our life force is running low, or when there are blocks in the body, we can experience stress, illness, negative emotions or pain.

What can reiki help with?

Reiki may sound quite woo-woo, but it is a great treatment for pregnancy because it is non-invasive, very safe and can be received even in early pregnancy when it can help with fatigue and nausea. It can also support fertility. Another reason it can be helpful during pregnancy is because it addresses your emotions as well as what is going on in your body. Pregnancy is often a time that brings up buried emotions or memories, and reiki is a gentle way of helping to release stress, fear, worry or doubts. Therapists describe the peace of mind you experience during a reiki session as creating mental space that helps you enjoy being pregnant and beginning to bond with your baby.

As well as creating a deep sense of calm and relaxation, reiki can have other benefits, including:

- Improving sleep and energy levels
- Helping with digestive issues, including nausea and heartburn
- Relieving aches and pains in the back and pelvis
- Relieving swollen, sore or restless legs
- Enabling the release of fears and anxieties
- Stabilising blood pressure
- Lessening side effects from medication
- Improving immunity
- Helping prepare for, or recovery from, surgery

A bonus is that because it is an energy-based therapy your baby will be included in the positive effects of the treatment. Mums often report their baby wriggling during a reiki session, and therapists say babies follow the therapist's hands during the treatments. Babies share the emotional chemistry of their mum during pregnancy so naturally they will enjoy tension and stress being replaced by a blissful warm relaxation. Reiki treatments can be given to babies once they are born, and they have been found to help babies sleep, which can come in handy!

Reiki FAQs

- **How long does a treatment last?** Treatments tend to be 30–60 minutes in length.
- **How many treatments do I need?** It is recommended to have a course of treatments, perhaps once a week or fortnight. The benefits will start straight away but increase over a series of treatments.
- **How can I find a good practitioner?** Word of mouth is always great – ask around for a recommendation. You might get a referral from another alternative practitioner such as a yoga teacher or massage therapist. Local natural-health clinics will often have a reiki practitioner. There are no academic qualifications for practising reiki – but you can ask whether the practitioner is level 1 or 2, or a reiki master. You can look for a practitioner who is a pregnancy or birth professional (perhaps as a doula, antenatal teacher or in another alternative therapy) so that they have a good understanding of pregnancy anatomy.

- **How much can I expect to pay?** Sessions are priced from £30 to £60 per hour depending on location and experience.

RELATIONSHIP

The responsibility of keeping a human being alive should never be under-estimated and it can place a strain on your relationship with your partner. It can cause anxiety, depression, short tempers and deep, abiding resentments. Factor in the modern-day problem of 'who is returning to work and when?', 'who does what at home?', 'who knows best?' when it comes to parenting and you can find yourself, one day, kneeling at the washing machine, looking back at your pre-baby life with a deep longing. You love your baby, but you can't even remember why you wanted a baby with your partner.

It is entirely normal to question yourself, your methods and those of your other half. Don't keep it all held in. I've known women ready to castrate their partner as he forgot, yet again, to restack the bottle steriliser, and dads who spend longer and longer at the office because at home they get nothing but criticised for things they seem to keep doing wrong.

Please cut each other a *lot* of slack in those first few months. Get as much help as you can afford – either in monetary terms or those of familial relations. The saying 'It takes a village to raise a child' should be 'It takes a village to raise a child *and* save a relationship.' Having just one uninterrupted hour with your partner to have a coffee out of the house while granny babysits can be completely reviving. Do not feel guilty about wanting to spend some time with the person you made the baby with – but without the baby. More than anything, the baby wants its parents to stay together. If that means they must go to the cinema without him, then so be it.

The chances are, you will instinctively nurture your baby. But you must also nurture your relationship. Your perspective can get all messed up in the first couple of years of a baby's life. I promise you, when they are sitting their GCSEs you will wonder why it mattered so much whether they took their daytime nap in a cot or a pram. I'm not belittling your best intentions or how important it is to be a good parent – I'm just saying that you might occasionally benefit from standing back, taking a deep breath and wondering whether some of the small shit really matters as much as it seems to. It is too easy to forget the biggest thing of all: staying in love with the one you once loved so much that you chose to start a new human with them.

Tips

- Don't presume your partner is psychic. State clear, reasonable expectations. If necessary, write them down and stick them on the fridge. This can be as simple as:

> **Please:**
>
> Empty nappy bin
> Buy milk and bread
> Tax car
> Kiss me!
> Cancel gym subscription
> Remember to kiss me

- Remain polite with each other. No grunting when you're handed a cup of tea. Smile and say thanks.

- Make eye contact. This sounds mental to someone without a baby. But you will spend so much time looking at your baby and thinking about its needs that you may go for days without looking into your partner's eyes. Eye contact is intimacy – it matters.

- Try to share a meal. This isn't easy with a baby, but a gentle evening routine from six to ten weeks should buy you an hour or two together at dinner time.

- Don't just talk about the baby. Swap other news – even if it's just the plot of a drama you watched on TV or a newspaper article you read.

- Articulate your feelings: good and bad. Try to use 'I' statements rather than 'you'; for example, 'I feel bad that you can't play golf this weekend, but I would love to spend some time with you' is so much better than, 'You can't play golf this weekend, you know! You need to be here with us!' Or 'You are always worrying about the baby and you never worry about me! You said you would make time to clear the spare room out this weekend but you never think about anyone but yourself!' Compare this to, 'I'm feeling a bit lost and needy. I could use some attention from you. And I would love it if we could use this weekend to clear the spare room.' When we hear 'You!' we can get easily riled and defensive.

- Laugh together – it's so damn easy to stop making each other laugh when you're tired and fed up. So, at least, watch a funny movie or comedy show together. It can be a great way of easing tension between you.

- Try to spend time with other couples in the same situation – this is one of the greatest long-term benefits of antenatal courses. Knowing everyone is feeling the same will lighten the mood and the load.

- Even if you don't fancy sex, remember to hold hands, cuddle and kiss each other. This gentle, physical intimacy is the glue that will hold you together.
- Remember that everything is a phase. Everything will pass.

■ RETURNING HOME – THE FIRST TWO WEEKS

Regardless of how your birth went, as a brand-new mum you will need time to rest and recover. If you didn't have a home birth, it's very special to bring your baby home. Hopefully, you return feeling excited and proud at your amazing achievement. Adrenalin will be your friend: keeping you going even if you haven't had much sleep over the previous couple of days. But, be warned – if you don't rest up in the first two weeks, you can crash and burn.

When you get home, get straight into your pyjamas and get into bed. Make the most of this glorious time. You will never have such a right to be pampered again (at least not until you have another baby and then, with another child to look after, you will look back on this time and wonder why you didn't eek out the relaxation for as long as you could).

Keep your baby close to you if you can – this will help establish breastfeeding or help closeness if bottle feeding.

Don't be tempted to jump up and do a supermarket shop, even if you feel well and energetic. Using the sporting analogy again, you've finished a marathon, you need to *rest* and *sleep* whenever you can.

I recommend that you:

- Stay in bed for the first week
- Stay near your bed for the second week

Your body is healing and needs to rest, be nurtured and not rushed back into action.

Remaining in your pyjamas is a very clever way of ensuring that guests don't stay too long. Child-free friends may not understand that you won't be providing lunch when they arrive with a huge present, delighted for you and keen to crack open the champagne. Entertaining is exhausting when you've had a baby – it's probably because half (or more) of your brain is preoccupied with your baby's well-being, and listening to outside gossip may feel oddly draining. This is OK – you will find who's-doing-what-to-whom-at work interesting again one day – it's just that your clever instincts to protect your young have (temporarily or permanently) altered your priorities overnight.

Having said that, fresh air and a break from central heating are good for babies (and you), so use any outdoor space that you have to sit with your feet up if the season allows. Of course, keep your baby's delicate skin well out of the sun and use a cotton hat and socks, as baby may get cool quite quickly, and make sure they are wrapped up warm in the colder months.

You will feed roughly every two hours to begin with – occasionally it will be after 90 minutes; sometimes you might get three hours between feeds. Sometimes a baby may go four hours without asking for a feed. Unless medically advised, this is nothing to worry about. Babies who are feeding well will be back to their birth weight after about 10–14 days. They should then put on about 6–8 ounces, or 180–240 grams, a week.

Practicalities

Getting your house in order – both literally and metaphorically – can make a huge difference to how you feel once baby arrives. Here is some stuff you might not have thought about.

Food for you

Stock up the freezer with meals before your baby arrives – you will need to eat and might find that you won't have the time (or the inclination) to cook. Friends will ask if you need anything. They really do mean it! Take up any offers of help.

High-protein/iron-rich foods (such as green vegetables and lamb) are good for replenishing your iron levels, which will inevitably have dropped after birth. You don't need to be following any sort of healthy-eating plan, but a varied diet and plentiful calories will do your milk supply no harm at all. Of course, even women who are genuinely malnourished manage to feed their babies, but your own energy levels will be aided by eating well.

Drink plenty of water – this is important if you're breastfeeding, but it will also aid the arrival of your slightly scary post-birth poos.

Guests and family

If you want guests, consider limiting them to mid-morning and mid-afternoon. This way you won't feel that you have to provide a meal. Politely ask them to liaise with your partner by phone/text prior to leaving to check it is still OK to come over. That may be your only time for a nap that day. This can feel mean-spirited, especially when friends are so keen to see you and the baby. But this is a time of self-preservation. If you're worried about upsetting anyone, tell a white lie and say that the midwife has instructed you to get some rest. Of course, loved ones can be wonderful to lift your mood if you're feeling a bit low – and never is a house happier and calmer than when a brand-new baby has arrived. But just be mindful of not over-doing the socialising at this early stage.

If you have complicated family dynamics, make a plan for who visits when before your baby arrives, but warn everyone that they may need to be flexible if you are unwell or tired. Emotions run high when babies arrive: in-laws who have always got along famously may suddenly become a little competitive. Try to let your partner deal with any dramas during these first few weeks. You won't get this time back. You won't want to look back on it as being unnecessarily stressful. Good communication is normally key to avoiding any meltdowns.

Social media has thrown up all sorts of new ways to upset people. Older generations may not understand your need to spread your happiness with the wider world before them, so consider how best to handle birth announcements. Grandparents are likely to become your greatest source of support in the next few years – don't piss them off over something as simple as a birth announcement.

Baby Practicalities

Clothes

New babies tend to wear a short-sleeved vest beneath a long sleeved Babygro. This gives two layers to hold any leaky nappies in place. Whether they need socks, cardigans and hats as well is all weather-dependent.

Their extremities will get cold, even in a warm house, which is why most Babygros cover feet. Their hands and feet will always feel quite cool – that's normal. If you suspect they are over-heating, feel the back of their neck and use a thermometer.

If you have a summer baby and it's *very* hot, they might be OK in just a nappy and vest. They can even sleep like that, loosely swaddled in a light blanket, on hot nights. Don't leave them directly in a breeze from an open window.

Your own body temperature does a good job of regulating theirs, so babywearing in a sling and co-sleeping is recommended for this. Many baby monitors now have temperature gauges and many parents find these very reassuring.

If you want to buy clothes for your baby before they are born, consider the season in which they will be a certain age/size. Millions have been wasted by mums falling in love with a three-to-six-month-size summer dress only to realise that when their baby is five months old it is zero degrees outside as it's January. Don't say I didn't warn you.

Where should my baby sleep?

Babies like to sleep with their mothers. This is pretty obvious if you think about it – they've heard your voice for months and you are the source of all milky warmth. Many studies have demonstrated that babies in the same room as mum (and possibly dad) cry less, sleep more and feed more easily. Many couples now choose the side-by-side cots, which attach to the bed, as they find this gives them the reassurance of having baby close by but also reduces any worry that co-sleeping in the same bed might harm their child.

The unfortunately named ISIS (Infant Sleep Information Service) is keen for parents to know that you mustn't be afraid of having your baby close to you while sleeping for the first six months. It provides free downloadable sheets containing the most up-to-date NICE guidelines to help you decide what is best for you. ISIS says:

A number of global studies have shown that babies sleeping in their parents' room have a lower risk of sudden infant death syndrome (SIDS) compared to babies sleeping in a separate room. The amount by which room sharing reduces the risk of SIDS is large. A study looking at SIDS cases in 20 locations across Europe estimated that 36 per cent of SIDS deaths could have been prevented if the baby had slept in a cot in the same room as the parents.

Like so much of this book – and so much of being a parent – your choices will depend on a balance between the way you view risk, what is best for your baby and what is best for you (and your family).

See **routine** (page 291) for thoughts on a routine for your baby.

Co-sleeping

Co-sleeping or bed-sharing has had a bad press in recent years, but when done safely, it can provide mum and baby with more quality sleep, and it can make breastfeeding easier. You will often find that first-time mums co-sleep less than those who already have children. With each subsequent baby, most mums find that by co-sleeping they get more rest. It is estimated that a fifth of all babies sleep with their parents for at least part of the night.

In 2014 NICE changed its guidance, downgrading the relationship between co-sleeping and sudden infant death syndrome from a 'risk' to an 'association'. In other words, co-sleeping does not cause SIDS but does appear in instances of it where risk factors occur. If bed-sharing suits you and your partner, take a few sensible precautions:

- Never put your baby between you and your partner. Place them at the side of the bed, but not too close to the edge.

You may want to put a rolled up towel on the side to stop your baby falling off (this isn't likely but may put your mind at rest). If the bed is next to a wall, make sure that baby is far enough away that they won't become wedged in the space.

- Sleep on your side with your baby close at chest level. Mums will often instinctively bend up their legs, which creates a safe space beside them.
- You and your partner mustn't drink alcohol and then have your baby in your bed.
- Keep your quilt and pillow away from your baby. They will get too hot. Use a thin, separate blanket for them.

Getting organised

New babies keep you shockingly busy. Being organised will truly help. Don't keep all nappy-changing equipment upstairs, or you'll spend the next two years running up and down stairs. Have a small, portable basket/box of nappy-changing gear to hand in the area you spend most time: probably the kitchen or living room. This will make it so much easier when granny offers to do a nappy change. You won't say, 'Upstairs, by the cot are the nappies, the Babygros are second drawer down – oh, don't worry, I'll do it myself.' Women are our own worst enemies at this. And grannies like to help.

Your changing basket should contain:

3 × nappies
1 packet wipes/cotton wool
Calendula oil for bottoms (such as Weleda – see Resources)
2 vests
2 Babygros
2 muslins

1 pair of socks
1 cardigan
Nipple cream
A handful of nappy bags

You can carry this basket up to bed at night and add a few snacks, some breast pads and a sports bottle of iced water for the long nights. Refilling the nappy basket is a great job for dad to do each morning if he has returned to work.

Your Physical Recovery

Bleeding

Whether you birth vaginally or by abdominal birth (**caesarean section** – see page 115), you will bleed for between two and six weeks. This is called lochia and is just your body getting rid of the lining of your uterus (womb) ready for another baby (yikes!). It may flow regularly or not, similar to a heavy period. It will become lighter as your uterus heals. You may notice small clots, but it will change to pink then brown, and eventually to yellow-white. If you try to do too much too soon, you will notice the lochia start to flow heavily again. Don't ignore this. Rest up. If your blood flow starts to look fresh again – bright red, rather than brown or pink – or you pass a clot any bigger than a 50-pence coin, call your hospital. It's a good idea to keep any clots on a sanitary towel, as the midwife will want to examine it for signs of retained placenta (I know, midwives do not get the credit they deserve!).

Stock up on maternity pads: 3 packs of 12 should do to start. Don't use tampons for the first six weeks after you have your baby, as this can introduce bacteria into your still-healing uterus, causing an infection. You may need to change your pad every hour or two to start with, then every three or four hours in the coming days and weeks. Always wash your hands before and after changing your pad.

Post-birth poo

This may be as terrifying as the birth itself. Don't rush it. If you don't go for a day or two, don't stress. You probably didn't eat much in labour and your body is very kind in allowing your lower regions to have a short break. Tearing to your back passage is – thankfully – extremely rare but, nevertheless, pushing a baby out puts a huge amount of pressure on your botty. It may ache and feel 'heavy' for several days afterwards. If possible, take a bath every day (showering won't do quite such a god job of cleaning inside) to keep your nethers clean and infection-free. Drink lots of water to keep your bowels hydrated, and eat healthy fruit and veggies. When you do need to 'go' it might help to hold loo roll or a pad onto your vagina and perineum while you patiently wait for nature to take its course. If you can't go, don't sit there straining. Get off, walk about a bit, drink more water and try again when you feel the party may be about to start.

Stitches/sore perineum

This is an actual conversation I overheard in a Manchester nail salon. It's a Saturday afternoon, the room is busy with women getting dolled up. Aromas of chemicals and coffee float above the pairs of heads bent over six nail stations. Nobody whispers. These women are frank, fearless and lethal with a nail file. A regular customer walks in to a chorus of coos with her two-day-old baby. She's getting her falsies done. The new mum sits in the raised waiting area, which is positioned just high enough that the entire shop will hear every word you say.

NAIL TECHNICIAN: How was it then, you know, the birth?

MUM: All right thanks. It's just birth isn't it? It was fine.

NAIL TECHNICIAN: Aww lovely. And how's your mum?

MUM: Oh, not bad, you know (lifting a cheek), just a couple of stitches.

[Filing stops and a quizzical s i l e n c e descends on the whole nail salon for five seconds.]

NAIL TECHNICIAN: Not yer *bum*! I said yer *mum*!

Unfortunately, not every woman feels the safe, trusting companionship of a northern nail shop to talk so openly about her derriere. But it's normal for your undercarriage to feel sore, bruised and swollen after birth – even if you haven't had stitches. The pain may be just inside your vagina as well as visible outside. The bad news is that it is likely to worsen from day one to three, and then it should improve. The more handling you have had internally (such as **forceps** – see page 54), the worse it will be.

Try to avoid putting too much pressure on the area through sitting upright for long periods. You'll probably want to lie down or sit slightly to one side, perhaps with cushions to aid your positioning.

If sitting down is impossibly painful, you could hire or buy an inflatable Valley Cushion, which forms a valley to stop any pressure on your painful parts.

Take ibuprofen and paracetamol at the recommended dosage to ease the pain. They are both safe during breastfeeding.

If you have had stitches, you'll need to keep them clean (to prevent infection) with a bath at least once a day. Use perfume-free soap, but no bubble baths or lotions. The area needs to dry off fully to help prevent the healing wound from breaking down before the stitches fully dissolve. Change your maternity pad regularly. Some mums like to add salt to their bath water. Do your pelvic-floor clenches (see page 269), as this will also promote perineal/stitches healing.

Make sure you don't let your bladder become too full at any time, as this could cause it to become distended. Of course, having a pee can really sting, so either empty your bladder in the shower or keep a jug beside the loo and use it to pour clean lukewarm water over yourself as you go. This will dilute the hormones and chemical in urine that make it so astringent and painful.

If your perineum is very sore, holding a bag of frozen peas wrapped in a clean muslin cloth to the area may offer some relief.

You can also take the homeopathic remedy arnica, to ease bruising.

Rest up

Newborn babies sleep a lot. This calm, peaceful stage is Mother Nature's way of letting you recover from the exertion of giving birth.

Even when they are feeding every two to three hours (day and night), try to grab 40 winks during the day when your baby is sleeping. This is not easy – the adrenalin keeping you alert and happy is hard to switch off. Being so 'unproductive' can also feel wrong to modern women: we see our sleeping baby as a good time to send that email or mop that floor – *stop!* Delegate as much as you can during this time. Your only priority is *you* and *your baby.*

Having said that, it can be almost impossible to nod off when you're worried that the baby will wake up at any second. You might find it easier to nap deeply if your partner takes your baby out of your room for a little while after she's been fed. Newborn babies are surprisingly noisy. Don't feel guilty about asking daddy – or whoever is helping you – to mind the baby in another room while you grab a much-needed snooze.

Baby's well-being

Breathing

Even if they aren't crying, babies snuffle, cough and grunt in their sleep. Their lungs contain fluid ingested before birth, and watching them bring this up can be absolutely terrifying if you aren't expecting it. Don't panic – just hold them and perhaps lean them forward and slightly downwards to aid the coughing or vomiting that they do to clear their pipes. Their airways will contain more of this fluid if they were born by abdominal birth – the compressions of the birth canal during a vaginal birth squeeze much of it out; however, if your baby ever seems to be genuinely struggling to breathe, dial 999 immediately.

Cord care

There will be a little stump of cord left with a plastic peg attached to it. This can be a shock if you aren't prepared for it. Leave the cord to dry out – it is simply rotting flesh (nice!), so don't bath your baby until the cord falls off in seven to ten days post-delivery. It can actually get a bit niffy once it's ready to fall off, but any redness or puss seeping from the join should be looked at by your midwife.

There is no real rule about whether your baby's nappy should cover the cord or not, but if you have a boy, make sure his willy is pointing downwards as they are very skilled at peeing all over themselves – and their cord stump.

The cord will eventually fall off – as a scab would. Don't be tempted to pick or pull it when it's nearly off. It needs to fully heal and you'll be left with a lovely belly button (interestingly, whether it's an inny or an outy is actually formed at conception rather than the clamping stage).

You can simply put the stump and the peg in the dustbin (take heed from *Sex and the City*'s Miranda who accidentally tossed her baby's cord in the air and the cat ran off to have it as breakfast).

Baby nails

It is tempting to cut baby's nails – they can be surprisingly long and they can scratch their faces in their sleep. But leave the scissors for now. You have years ahead of bartering your child with biscuits to get them to have their nails cut. Instead, a little petroleum jelly or nipple cream, such as Weleda (see Resources) (which you may have lying around to keep your nipples peachy) on the ends magically softens and dissolves any extra-long bits. Never bite them, no matter how tempting it is! This can cause little, painful 'wicks' along the sides of the nails, which can become paronychia – a nail infection that would require local antibiotics.

Cleaning your baby

Babies do not get dirty, and it is recommended that you leave the white **vernix** covering to be absorbed naturally into their skin (see page 316).

If they were overdue, their skin might be very dry, so bathing them at this stage will only make their skin drier. But it's really important to clean in all your baby's little creases around the neck and the bottom. These can quite quickly get sore from moisture – milk, vomit, wee and so on. Use warm water and cotton wool to wash around their face: gently tip their head back to squeeze water from the cotton wool into the folds of the neck and pat dry with a soft towel. Wash bottoms by lying the baby flat on a towel or changing mat, and separate any tightly folded flesh with your fingers – again, squeeze a wet cotton-wool ball with lukewarm water across the area and pat dry thoroughly. (For a very mild cleanser, see the Weleda entry in Resources.)

Once the cord falls off after seven to ten days, you can enjoy bathing them (see **Weeks two to four, bathing** on page 321).

Sudden infant death syndrome

This is not a happy topic to write about in a book that celebrates the miracle of birth, but, as always, knowledge is power, and there is a lot you can do to minimise the small risk that your baby won't survive their first year. From 700,000 births, just less than 300 babies die unexpectedly in the UK each year. Boys are slightly more likely to die from SIDS (formerly called 'cot death'); premature or low birth-weight babies are more at risk. Those whose mothers smoked during and after pregnancy are also at greater risk. SIDS usually occurs when a baby is asleep, although it can occasionally happen while they're awake.

Nobody knows exactly why SIDS occurs, but one, or a combination of factors, is normally present. According to the NICE guidelines, in the first year of a child's life you should *not*:

- Place a baby on their front or side to sleep.
- Have a smoker in the house.
- Allow an adult to sleep with a baby on the sofa or in a chair.
- Allow an adult who has recently consumed alcohol or taken drugs to sleep with your baby.
- Co-sleep with a baby who has a low birth weight.
- Co-sleep with a baby who was born prematurely.
- Let your baby get too hot or too cold. Some monitors have room thermometers and can help make sure the temperature is between 16°C and 20°C.

This means that you should:

- Always place your baby on their back to sleep.
- Place your baby towards the end of their cot, Moses basket or pram. This allows air to circulate around the head to regulate their temperature.
- Make sure that their head is not covered by a blanket or a sleeping bag that rides up and over their face. A normal blanket should be tucked in no higher than their shoulders.
- Let your baby sleep in a cot or Moses basket in the same room as you for the first six months.
- Use a mattress that's firm, flat, waterproof and in good condition.
- Breastfeed your baby.

Health visitor and Red Book

The health visitor (HV) makes contact between 10 and 14 days to arrange a birth visit at your home. They will bring or go through the little NHS Red Book that you were given in the hospital. It is worth reminding your HV if you didn't get one at the hospital. This book will detail all your child's immunisations, growth measurements and screenings until they are five years old. Take it to every doctor/HV appointment regarding your baby. It is probably worth carrying it in your nappy bag for the first few weeks in case of emergencies.

(See also **health visitor** page 193.)

Help at home

The help that you arrange to ease your transition into life as a mummy is a very personal choice that depends on how much family/community help you will get, how confident you are about caring for a new baby and your budget.

The best support for a new mum is a close, entirely sane female relative who moves into the guest cottage in the garden from where she sensitively and discreetly meets your needs, preparing nutritious meals, helping with breastfeeding, changing the sheets while you're in the bath and showing you how to expertly wind your little munchkin. There is no ego battle; no tricky past between you and your husband adores her. But obviously, we are talking about the real world here.

Granny If you are lucky enough to have your own mother around and willing to help, they are a godsend in the first few weeks. They love you and your baby and have already seen you in various states of undress throughout your life, so you may be less self-conscious learning to breastfeed in front of them.

New grandchildren are an amazing way of healing rifts between mothers and daughters, so even if you have a tricky relationship with her now, keep an open mind about how you might work together once baby arrives.

Try to be clear about your needs. Don't expect her to be psychic. If your mum is nervous about doing everything 'wrong', reassure her that you are grateful for her support, and if she doesn't do everything exactly the way you want, don't sweat it. You have decades of raising your children ahead, so let little differences of opinion slide in the first few weeks.

If you have a spare room, you might wish to discuss if she wants to move in for a few days once your partner has gone back to work (or before). I couldn't have coped without my mum in the first few weeks of my baby's lives (or now actually!) and I never loved her more than when she would creep in my room and take a baby grizzling with a wet nappy at 6am so I could get another hour's sleep.

Mother-in-law Now, don't laugh, if – like me – you're lucky enough to have married a man with a kind and big-hearted mum, you will also find that she is a marvel when you have a baby. Mums-in-law tend to be a bit more worried about 'treading on toes' or imposing themselves on your new family, but there is no reason why they shouldn't be an important part of your baby's life. Grandparents offer wonderful gifts of knowledge, fun and life experience to your children. Keep them close if you possibly can – they can be your greatest allies in the years of parenting that lie ahead. It's hard to imagine right now, but there will come a time when you and your partner want to stay overnight at a friend's wedding and you will thank God that you have grandparents who love him as much as you do as you hand over his overnight bag.

Postnatal doulas (see page 150) will help you get to know your baby and help with everything from breastfeeding to nappy changing. But they will also do light housework and cooking. Discuss exactly what you think you might need, and listen to their advice. Most postnatal doulas do not sleep at your home but visit during the day at a convenient time.

Maternity nurses are expensive but can be extremely valuable, especially if you don't have family nearby and are nervous about caring for a newborn. It is normally best to find one on recommendation. Maternity nurses are not medically trained – although they should have an up-to-date First Aid qualification (that has not been done online) and be CRB checked. They tend to focus on looking after the baby – so be careful that they aren't pushing your little one in the sunshine while you're at home hanging out wet Babygros! You also need to consider how you and your partner will feel about having someone else living in your home for a few weeks – if it's unusual for you to be sharing a kitchen with someone you don't know while in your dressing gowns at 7am, this may not be your preferred option. A good maternity nurse knows that you are the mother and won't patronise you. I've heard tales of maternity nurses rearranging baby's bedrooms without permission or, on one occasion, a maternity nurse gave a breastfed baby its first bottle of formula without the mum's permission. Set out your expectations clearly.

Cleaner If you're the sort of person who is happier in a tidy house, living among new-baby chaos can be a challenge. If you already have a cleaner, don't be tempted to cancel them while you're on maternity leave – one the greatest ways of easing baby blues is a brisk walk with a pram while someone else cleans the kitchen. If your budget doesn't allow for outside help, discuss how you and your partner might divide the domestic chores now that you have a baby. Don't feel guilty about finding the domestic workload overwhelming – you have a baby to raise!

Emotions

How you feel in the first few weeks is likely to be affected by how you feel about the birth. Don't be **shut up!** (see page 306) by that old sentiment, 'You've got a healthy baby and that's what matters.' It's not OK to be told that your birth experience is irrelevant. Talk about it. Don't bottle it up. Tell your **health visitor** (see page 193) and visiting midwife what happened, and if you have any questions about the birth itself, be sure to ask them. If you don't get a satisfactory response, seek out help. Cry if you need to, celebrate and cheer, and spread the positivity if you need to! Just don't feel you can't express your feelings. Women do other women no favours when we pretend things are better (or worse) than they really are.

On day three or four post-birth you will have a mood slump. This is normal and will probably pass. It's your hormones levelling out and it is likely to coincide with your milk supply coming in and possibly giving you sore boobs (see **breastfeeding**, page 78). You may feel tearful and tired and in need of a lot of cuddles from your partner and your baby. Hunker down, read a good book or watch some TV, and be kind to yourself.

If you find that you can't stop crying or are feeling extremely lethargic over a few days or having any sort of dark and distressing thoughts about hurting yourself or your baby, tell your midwife, health visitor or GP. Postnatal depression is on the rise, and support is available if you – or someone on your behalf – can seek it out (see Resources).

S is for ...

SEX

Ahhh – I am so in awe of you pregnant women in your glorious fecundity, fresh from the nooky factory. Making a baby with another human being is life's greatest (free) hobby. Even if your journey has been fraught with the emotion of infertility, you've hopefully picked up this book because all has worked out well. Now, you too are staring down the barrel of a life in which fatigue, bed-sharing and sick-splattered nighties will put paid to your sex-life –because it's the world's greatest irony that the little buggers are likely to put pressure on any such shenanigans for several years forthwith. You know by now that I prefer to be optimistic, so here's the take-home: make the most of this very special time together.

I don't mean that pregnancy will necessarily be the time to start extending your sexual repertoire: those ever-so-appealing swingers' parties with the octogenarian neighbours can wait. But staying connected as a couple is worth prioritising. Impending parenthood can feel overwhelming and terrifying: try to hold onto each other – literally and metaphorically – to ensure you land softly on the other side.

The early days

Having said the above, go easy on the love-making in the first 12 weeks of pregnancy. Female orgasms can dislodge and destroy a newly developing embryo. It's all a bit delicate in there at first, so demonstrate adoration to your partner through other, less, er, impactful means. I mean, c'mon, you got pregnant in the first place – you don't need blow-by-blow instructions!

There's a very good chance that sex is the last thing on your mind in the first trimester, what with the sickness, sore boobs, a crampy belly and bone-crushing fatigue – not to mention the absence of booze, which may well have played a significant role in your pre-pregnancy couple-push-ups.

The second and third trimesters

You might find that your sex drive simply doesn't resurface at all in pregnancy. Don't give yourself a hard time; you're growing a baby – you've got a lot on!

Or you might find that your hormones kick in during the second and third trimester, and not having to hold your belly in for the first time in your adult life brings a new type of bedroom liberation.

And just think: for perhaps the first time ever, you don't have even the slightest niggle in the back of your mind about getting pregnant. You already smashed that one into the back of the net! And don't worry about there being any negative effect on your pregnancy once it is well established. Your funny little baba is tucked up in his secure sleep-sack completely oblivious to how much work you're putting into your relationship for the sake of his stable future.

Of course, that epic belly bump and possible aching joints might mean that you need to get creative with positions and cushions. Listen to your body as always and, if it hurts, it's probably a bad idea (there will never be a market for *Fifty Shades of Grey: The Maternity Months*).

Before the birth

Of course, sex is apparently good at bringing on labour naturally (see **induction – natural methods**, page 215). But don't be fiddling about in your lady cave once your waters have gone. You need to keep the area free from any potential germs, and no willy is yet to earn an EU Blue Flag.

(For information on sex after baby, see **Postnatal/baby check** page 330).

SHUT UP!

This is the worst thing to say someone who is angry, upset or confused. And yet, how often have you heard the phrase 'You have a healthy baby and that's what matters' uttered to a new mum? It is tantamount to telling her to shut up. It's never meant maliciously; it beseeches the mother to look on the bright side, thank her blessings and feel grateful. And forward-thinking optimism is extremely useful as a mum. But it fails to recognise that a woman with a brand-new baby may need to talk, cry, shake with anger, scream for answers and roar at the moon about the birth she has just experienced.

Even after the most life-affirming, joyous births imaginable, new mums need to talk it through. Ever noticed how women tell their birth stories in minute detail? The step-by-step chronology, pauses, deep breaths, repetition, a few laughs and maybe even a few shudders? That's what we need to do. We need to process the event we just went through and to try to make some frickin' sense of it.

But it can be so hard to discuss. Some listeners can be over-sensitive, wondering if you're depressed or struggling to bond. You worry that they will gossip that you aren't coping. You may not want sympathy or applause – you just need to talk.

Who can I talk to?

Independent midwife (see page 212) Even if you did not have one for your birth, you might like to obtain your notes and talk through what happened with an independent midwife (IM). They will be impartial but also possess a clinical understanding of the story. They can explain what happened, why and whether it would be inevitable again. Obtaining NHS notes can cost around £50, and the IM will also charge a one-off fee for their time.

A birth crisis helpline There are several groups on social media that offer peer-to-peer support. The Birth Trauma Association can be found on Facebook and is extremely knowledgeable (see Resources).

Doula (see page 150) Find one who is specifically trained in postnatal debriefs. They will be a supportive ear but won't have a full clinical understanding of events and may not be able to fully empathise with the hospital protocols that may have been operating at the time of your birth; however, they can be a godsend and immensely supportive.

Your antenatal group The 'me too!' stories might be just what you need to feel less alone.

Your partner This won't be ideal in every case, as they may also be processing the experience in their own way. They may view the birth differently. Don't be discouraged if they don't share your same anxiety about the birth. It doesn't mean that you are 'wrong'. It's probably good therapy to find the humour in what you went through together. Laughter is a great healer and if you can eventually see the funny side of the experience, that's no bad thing.

Your midwife You can also ask to go over your notes with your midwife, and they can help you put your labour memories into a more chronological order. This may be done more formally at around six weeks after the birth, at your request.

Postnatal depression (PND – see Resources) is on the increase, however, so don't be afraid to express your thoughts to your GP or health visitor if you are feeling consistently down, view yourself as a failure or have thoughts of hurting yourself or your baby. These are warning signs that must not be ignored.

▪ SKIN

For the first time in 15 years you can finally stop holding your stomach in, your hair is glossy and your boobs are luscious, but – if you're unlucky – your skin is breaking out in teenage spots. It doesn't happen to all women during pregnancy: some find their skin has never been better thanks to plentiful oestrogen. But other hormones, including testosterone, create more oil and can clog up pores in which bacteria multiply rapidly. If you are genuinely worried by painful, unprecedented acne that emerges rapidly, speak to your doctor. Sadly, there is little that they can do because most oral or topical acne medications are not recommended in pregnancy. Even over-the-counter creams that contain beta-hydroxy acid (BHA) and salicylic acid have not been studied in pregnant women, so it's up to you whether you want to take the small risk that they might be absorbed through the skin. The more serious drugs that cause birth defects include Accutane, Retin-A and other topical retinoids, including tretinoin, isotretinoin, tazarotene and adapalene. Read the label. Basically, if you can't spell it, don't use it.

What *can* you use?

Fear not. Most breakouts during pregnancy can be treated with over-the-counter skincare products: use a non-comodogenic tinted moisturiser with SPF (see Resources) and a decent cleanser with water – especially at the end of the day when it helps to take off your day's make-up or city grime as soon as you're behind closed doors.

Having struggled with blocked pores and zits over the years, I've now discovered an amazing all-natural gel containing vitamin B_3 (niacinamide), aloe vera and witch hazel called Metazene

5, which is available from America (see Resources). In tests, 82 per cent of acne sufferers saw a marked improvement using niacinamide in eight weeks, and it is fast becoming a buzzword in dermatology circles. You heard it here first.

And perhaps use a chemical–manual scrub three times a week (see Resources): leave it on while you clean your teeth and rinse it off with a gentle rub. It will help to slough away the skin cells and oil that are blocking the pores.

And just think, when you're breathing your baby out or waiting for your caesarean, one more motivation will be knowing that your skin will almost immediately get better.

Hormone fluctuations after birth may continue to affect your skin for years, so get to know your cycle via the fantastic Hormone Horoscope website (see Resources).

STILLBIRTH

This is not a pleasant topic in a book about birth, but every woman wants to know steps she might take to avoid a stillbirth. It's also paramount to know that even in the awful event of learning that your baby has died in utero, you still have choices. A stillbirth is classified as a baby that has ceased to live after 24 weeks gestation. If a baby dies during pregnancy it is called an 'intra-uterine' stillbirth, or a death that occurs during labour is called an 'intra-partum' stillbirth. Prior to 24 weeks it is termed a miscarriage. There are five stillbirths in every 1,000 births in the UK. More than half of these are 'unexplained', but contributing factors in the remainder include genetic abnormalities, prematurity and birth trauma.

If it is apparent that a baby has failed to survive pregnancy, the woman may be advised to have labour induced immediately or to wait to see if labour occurs naturally. She can wait as long as there is no threat to her own life. She can still request the type of birth that she feels is right for her. Some women stick to their original plan of a home birth, some opt to be induced and others may demand a caesarean section. This last option will be advised against due to the long- and short-term risks to mum. But if a woman really cannot face labour knowing that her baby is deceased, I say she should have a fully informed right to an abdominal birth.

How to minimise your risk of a stillbirth:

- Do not smoke, use drugs or drink alcohol.
- Maintain a healthy weight before and during pregnancy.
- Monitor your baby's movements.
- Report any stomach pain or vaginal bleeding without delay.
- Avoid certain foods (see **diet**, page 140).
- Attend all your antenatal appointments.

There are some wonderful charities supporting couples who experience stillbirth (see Resources). These days it is normal for parents to be encouraged to photograph, hold and even dress or bathe their stillborn babies. Research suggests that this helps many heartbroken couples to move forward with the bereavement process.

STRETCH MARKS

These are a potentially irritating and itchy side effect of pregnancy that arise from your skin strettttccccchhhhing over your growing bump, ballooning boobs and possibly widening back and expanding thighs.

You can't prevent stretch marks, but they might be moderately eased by keeping yourself and your skin hydrated and moisturised (see Weleda in Resources for suggestions). It can be very helpful to apply a good lotion or oil at least once a day all over your body. Making sure you avoid putting on excessive weight in pregnancy through good **diet** and **exercise** (see pages 140 and 162) can help to minimise your chance of getting stretch marks; however, that shouldn't really be your main reason for staying fit and healthy.

After all, lines upon your skin, which denote your transition to becoming a mum, are nothing to be ashamed of. Some women may feel self-conscious in the longer term if the marks don't fade as much as they would like. It's hard to say whether expensive laser treatment actually works in reducing their severity, but that is the only option available today for women who aren't comfortable with the way stretch marks appear.

Give it time – you might be surprised by how much they fade over the passage of time. Or, wear them with pride like the sexy tigress that you are.

SWOLLEN FEET

This is one of those 'comedy' pregnancy ailments that is funny for everyone except the sufferer. We retain fluid in pregnancy, our veins are sluggish due to the hormone relaxin, and some swelling around the feet or ankles is pretty common. For most women it is largely harmless and can be eased by making sure you drink plenty of water, that you elevate your legs when sitting or lying, drink nettle tea, do some light exercise and avoid spending long periods of time standing up.

Nevertheless, swollen feet can be a very important sign of the serious condition pre-eclampsia, so do not delay in getting yourself seen by a doctor if your feet or lower legs swell up. The doctors will check your urine and blood pressure, and monitor you very carefully. If pre-eclampsia is diagnosed, they will discuss your options with you. If not – as long as it is completely ruled out – you can return to the list of measures above and send your partner in my direction if he laughs at your elephant feet.

SYMPHYSIS PUBIS DYSFUNCTION (SPD)

Sometimes called pubic symphysis joint pain, this can be a very painful condition of pregnancy caused by the hormone relaxin, which loosens your joints and renders your pelvic girdle less stable where the pubic bones meet at the front. The pain is caused by friction between the joints. A physiotherapist with expertise in women's health is your best source of help, as SPD relates to muscles and joints.

This is the advice suggested by physiotherapist Hannah Cooksey.

Hannah Cooksey on managing and minimising the risk of developing SPD

- Avoid parting your knees or standing on one leg.
- Get in and out of a car with your knees together.
- When turning in bed, keep your knees together and pull your tummy tight.
- Avoid crossing your legs and sitting cross-legged on the floor.
- Sit to dress the lower half of your body instead of standing on one leg.

- Don't put all your weight through one leg when, for example, standing in a shopping queue.
- Avoid carrying heavy things on one side of your body, such as carrying a bag over your shoulder or a child on one hip.
- Change the way you take the stairs (only if having problems) – do one step at a time or try going up or down sideways.

Exercise: knee squeezes (to relieve pubic symphysis pain)

Sit or lie with your knees bent, with a rolled towel between your knees, then squeeze for a few seconds. Repeat ten times. This will help to realign your pubic symphysis joint.

T is for ...

TENS MACHINE

This is a nifty little bit of pain-relieving kit with no side effects. Its name is an acronym for transcutaneous electrical nerve stimulation, so you can see why 'TENS' caught on.

A TENS machine is a small, battery-operated device that connects to your lower back in labour through sticky pads containing electrodes. When the machine is turned up, small electrical impulses are delivered to the body, which you might feel as a tingling sensation. The impulses can reduce the pain signals going to the spinal cord and brain, helping to take the edge off any pain and relaxing your muscles. There is also a belief that the impulses stimulate endorphins – your very own natural painkillers.

Clinical trials are ongoing, so for now you can take the word of countless women who have used them to good effect.

If nothing else, they are a great distraction and a way of communicating with your care provider without having to speak. They will simply watch you press a button with your thumb, which activates the impulses at the sign of each contraction.

How to use it

To get the most benefit from TENS, it's important that the settings are adjusted correctly for you and that you get started with it in early labour, as it seems to have a cumulative effective.

Make sure you don't cover your back in body lotion when you get out of the shower when in labour, as this will stop the pads from sticking. Once they are attached in the correct positions as explained in the leaflet, turn on the TENS machine to the lowest setting. You'll feel a slight tingling sensation pass through your skin. If it's uncomfortable, turn it down. The beauty of TENS is that *you* control its use and can gradually increase the strength of the settings.

Obviously, you can't use a TENS in a birth pool. But women who want a natural birth and are being well cared for often graduate from TENS to the water when things progress.

U is for ...

UTERUS

Your uterus is the amazing bag that grows with your baby and keeps it safe and snug. It is just a massive muscle plugged tightly shut at your cervix that has the ability to contract all by itself to gently release your baby into the world. Hidden, but awesome.

V is for ...

VERNIX

This is the white, creamy substance that covers your baby when it emerges into the world. It is odourless and contains nothing but goodness for their skin. It will seep in fairly quickly and shouldn't be washed off within the first two weeks.

W is for ...

WATER BIRTH

What do you think of when you think of water birth? Here are some common responses:

- 'I worry that the baby will drown.'
- 'I don't like water much, so it wouldn't be for me.'
- 'I desperately want a water birth. It's all I want!'
- 'I'd really like one, but the pool might not be available.'

Whatever your position on water births during your pregnancy, remember to keep an open mind. Some women have their heart set on a water birth but unexpectedly decide in labour that it's not for them, especially at the pushing stage. Others simply can't countenance the notion of being in water, but suddenly develop gills in labour and refuse to get out of their watery cocoon. There are, however, few topics more likely to receive an evangelical response than asking a woman who has had a successful water birth what it was like. They glaze over and look wistful – when it goes right, it can be like glimpsing heaven.

Water supports your whole body, which can be lovely when you feel like a sea cow unable to get comfortable on dry land. There is a freedom of movement that comes in a pool, and this allows you to sway about, kneel, lean and do whatever it is sea cows do to feel relaxed.

They offer privacy. Women often say that they don't want their husbands to be at the 'business end' so would prefer to be on a bed. Strangely, in a pool you actually have more privacy and can position yourselves in any way that you both feel most comfortable with. Dads often sit by the pool, forehead-to-forehead with mum who kneels on all-fours with arms over the edge of the bath.

Nobody can fiddle with you during labour when you are in a deep pool unless they are happy to get very wet themselves. So they have to ask you to move, to come over to them or change position. This gives the labouring woman complete control over her environment.

Water birth – all you need to know

Do hospitals offer pools to all birthing women? Yes – as long as there is availability. Almost all units now have pools, but sometimes there are practical issues that mean the pool is not available. All birth centres have pools and are less likely to be in use, so if a water birth is important to you, opting to labour there is a very smart move.

I want a home birth. Will my midwife bring a pool? Some private midwives have their own pools. You simply have to buy a fresh liner that is disposed of. If not, hire or buy one online (see Resources).

Where can I put a pool in my house? Ideally on the ground floor, as you don't know how good your joists are, and nobody wants to start birthing in their bedroom and finish up in the lounge surrounded by ceiling rubble. You simply need a hose and attachment for the taps (or mixer tap) and a good hot-water system. If you don't have continuous hot water, you can always part-fill, put the cover on the pool and wait for the tank to fill again. Labours are not quick. You should have time, but start the process of filling it when labour has begun.

Will the water be very warm? This won't be your concern. Your care provider will make sure that the water temperature is around 32–38°C. But trust yourself – tell your midwife if you are uncomfortably hot or cold.

Won't my baby breathe underwater? A baby does not take their first breath until they are born and stimulated with their head in the open air. It's important that nobody stimulates the baby into breathing before the rest of the body is delivered. You should be encouraged to keep your bottom underwater while the baby is born completely. Or, if you do lift your bum above the water once the head is out, your midwife should then ensure that you don't dip back down, in case the cold air has stimulated your baby to breathe. This sounds more complicated than it is. Your midwife will help you.

When can I get in the pool? This is a matter of some debate. A bath at home, in very early labour, can be restful and relaxing, and delays you arriving at the hospital too soon; however, once you are in well-established labour (at around, say, 5–6cm dilated) some women find that a labour that was progressing well slows right down in the water. This could be because walking and being upright was creating more efficient contractions – especially with a first birth. Many women will float horizontally in the pool, which feels lovely, but can have a similar effect to lying on your back on the bed.

It's also worth remembering that if you're hoping to avoid an epidural and go drug-free, the water might be your best form of pain relief. So, like all 'drugs' it might be best to wait until you are finding it hard to cope without it. But if not, enjoy the pool before you are ready for an epidural.

How will the midwife know I'm OK? He will monitor your baby's heartbeat every few minutes using an underwater Doppler. If the heart rate does raise any concerns, it is very easy for you to shift positions in the water so that they can listen in from a different angle. If your labour has slowed down too much, or there is some other cause for concern, you might be asked to get out of the pool to be checked. Sometimes, being back on dry land can change the baby's position for the better. Skilled midwives can see how dilated you are by using the 'purple line' method – this line appears in the coccyx area and becomes more defined with each centimetre of dilation.

What happens if I need the loo? The beauty of giving birth in the pool is that you don't have to go anywhere to use the loo! Wee is invisibly diluted into the water and poo is quickly and odourlessly sieved away into a receptacle (possibly a bin bag) by a midwife or a very helpful partner. Given that pooing and weeing in front of an audience is a very common birth anxiety, water birth is a brilliant way of avoiding any embarrassment.

Will the pool look very gory? Before the placenta is delivered, there will be a little **blood** (see page 76) (and possibly a little poo that didn't quite make it into the sieve) but I promise that nobody will care about that. A little blood can look like a lot in water, so don't be startled if it looks excessive.

What about the placenta? Not many midwives will be happy delivering the placenta in the pool, so you will probably get out to simply squat or lie on the necessary waterproof sheet with a towel around you, and the midwife will dispose of the placenta in a bed pan or similar. Discuss this with your midwife beforehand.

Who can't have a water birth? Some units will try to discourage women from having a water birth if they have some risk factors, including twins, a high body mass index (BMI) or a previous abdominal birth (**caesarean section** – see page 115). But, of course, some women with all these conditions could safely give birth in water. If you are met with resistance, discuss your options with your medical team and ask for support from your supervisor of midwives. You might find that an **independent midwife** (see page 212) will happily support your water birth choice if NHS protocol won't.

WEEKS TWO TO FOUR: LOOKING AFTER YOU AND YOUR BABY

I don't want to be a harbinger of doom, but this can be a tough time for new mums. If your partner took a couple of weeks off work, by week three they are likely to be heading back in again every morning, leaving you feeling a little vulnerable. You might not quite feel like making arrangements to meet friends for coffee or leaping around your local high street showing off your new baby. So you may feel a bit lonely and isolated. The adrenalin that sustained you for the first two weeks is probably waning a little, and the desire to sleep for more than two hours at a time may have become all-consuming. This period of time can feel worse if it's the middle of winter and you can't even enjoy a few minutes of fresh air sitting on the back step in your nightie. I'm really selling this, aren't I?

Ways to feel better organised

Set yourself realistic goals for each day. This may be little more than getting yourself and your baby washed and dressed. If you're really over-achieving, you might manage to do an online food delivery or cook a meal. Expect to be constantly interrupted and feel as though you are walking through mud. When you're at home all day, you won't believe how many Amazon deliveries you will accept on behalf of all your neighbours who are at work.

This is a great time to ask your mum or mum-in-law to stay for a few days, as long as you feel sure that you won't be hosting. Be clear that you would appreciate the help, and possibly set a flexible routine; for example, would they be happy taking your baby for a walk in the pram after its mid-morning feed? This would give you a chance to either have a nap or a shower and to throw the dirty laundry in the machine. Maybe they could cook the evening meals (it doesn't have to be dinner-party standard), or collect that parcel that is waiting for you at the sorting office? Even if you are grumpy and tired, try to express your gratitude sincerely when anyone helps. Raising a baby is a team effort from which everyone benefits – trust me, your support network will be priceless in the coming years.

Just because your partner is back at work, doesn't mean that they can't continue to be practical and helpful: can they possibly fix you a sandwich to leave in the fridge for lunchtime? (I can hear you laughing at how ridiculous that sounds now, but trust me, you're about to enter a world in which time is completely fucked up). Can they repack the changing basket with fresh Babygros, and so on? Or renew the house/car insurance, which is about to run out?

Try to get out of the house once a day – even if it's just to post a card in the box around the block. You can feel a bit caged-up at this point, so leaving the house is a good mood-enhancer. One Happy Birth Club mum had a real downer at this point (which was no surprise, as she had twins) so Pam prescribed that grandma came round and sat in the cafe next door to the hairdressers with the babies while the new mum went in and got a blow-dry. It was exactly what she needed and she came out feeling like herself again. This probably sounds unbelievably trivial. But it wasn't. All that this new mum needed was a short breather with a coffee and a magazine, and to get her hair washed. If it's something that is important to you, don't ignore the nagging sensation to do something that makes you happy.

Expressing

If you are breastfeeding and your supply is well established, this can be a good time to start expressing so that dad can do an evening feed. It is not for everyone and shouldn't be considered if you're struggling to produce enough milk. But, if you can feed from one breast in the morning when your milk is plentiful (say, at 7am) and simultaneously express from the other boob, that expressed milk can be put in the fridge.

Then feed as normal throughout the day. In the evening, you can do your last breastfeed at roughly 7.30–8pm – baby's bedtime – and go to bed yourself. This leaves dad to do the last feed of the day (or first of the night) at about 10.30–11pm. This means that you can sleep through until 2 or 3am, when you will do the middle-of-the-night feed. Although this can feel like the worst time to wake up, it's vital to keep this feed going from the breast, as your prolactin is highest at this time and needs to be stimulated to keep your supply going throughout the day.

It may be that your baby's latch is still a bit inconsistent at this stage, so don't rush to delegate this job if you do want to carry on breastfeeding. But this system can be a lifesaver if you are dying for some good-quality sleep, and it also means dad is intrinsically involved even if he has gone back to work. (See also **expressing/ pumping** on page 78.)

Emotions

Don't be surprised if you miss your old life/resent the confinement/hate your partner. This is normal and will not last forever. This time spent with a newborn baby can feel like treading water. Where once by 11am we would have been dressed up smart and planning lunch with colleagues, with our newborns we find ourselves wanting to crawl back under the duvet at 10am and eating cornflakes for dinner at 9pm. Our clothes don't fit, our careers feel desperately uncertain, and that's normally the point at which your partner will say that he's heading out to 'wet the baby's head' (again).

This can feel like torture. This *is* torture! Meanwhile, someone who popped their baby out five minutes ago appears on the red carpet to pick up her award for 'mother of the year' and you wonder what the hell you have done and why everyone seems to be better at it than you.

Just being present and unproductive is very difficult for most modern women. In our busy world, we often feel as if we have to be doing, rather than being; we have to have some kind of output to show for our time. Our brains are big and busy and are simply not used to the domestic drudgery of being at home all day with a baby that needs us and the ceaseless list of mind-numbing jobs that constantly require our attention.

Historically, and in some other cultures today, women are worshipped for their ability to birth, particularly in the first few weeks, and are encouraged to do absolutely nothing but hold, feed and love their baby. In China, this time is called the Golden Month. I don't exactly envy these women – I'd go insane with boredom if I wasn't allowed to leave the house, send work emails and keep one eye on my future as a human being that isn't 'just' a mother. But the idea of chilling the heck out for a while is a very good one, so make sure you enjoy this precious time – even if that means calling in extra help to get you through.

The friends you meet on your antenatal courses will sustain you in this time. The 'me too!' messages go a long way towards eradicating a sense of isolation, and the shared jokes will keep you smiling.

Bathing

One of the best things about this stage is finally being able to bath your baby. Hopefully, the cord stump has dried and fallen off and all the lovely vernix has been absorbed by their skin.

Bath time can become a fun and relaxing ritual for all of you. At this stage you will still only need to bath them two or three times a week; although particularly messy nappies might demand a good botty wash to stop skin getting sore.

Bathing your baby for the first time can be a bit nerve-wracking. You might want to have someone with you, not least to pass you the thing that you forget – until you get into a routine, you'll probably find this is a common occurrence!

Handling a wriggling, wet and slippery baby takes practice and confidence, but you and your baby will get used to bath time and start to enjoy it. Most babies find warm water soothing, and a bath might help a fussy baby to relax and calm down.

When should I bath my baby?

Choose a time of day when you're not expecting any interruptions and have time to devote to your baby. It's much better if your baby is awake and contented before you start and isn't in need of a feed.

When your baby is newborn you might find it easiest to bath him in the morning after a feed but before the morning nap – particularly if you have had lots of dirty nappies in the night or he has been quietly sick into the folds of his neck. Keeping this skin clean and dry is essential to avoid rashes and painful sores developing.

Warm water can help to relax your baby and make them sleepy. It's also a great job for other family members to help with. Dads often enjoy taking care of bath time and can share a bath with their baby. This is a lovely way for them – or you – to have precious skin-to-skin time with your quickly developing baby.

Where should I bath my baby?

At first, you might find it easier to use a sink or a small plastic baby bath placed inside your bath or on the tray beneath the shower.

Of course you can use your big bath, but it can be awkward, as you need to kneel or lean over the side. A specially made baby bathing seat or support may help. But never, ever leave your baby alone in the bath, no matter how secure they may seem in a bath seat. Tragedies can happen in a split second, so don't be lulled into thinking that you have time to run and grab the cotton wool that you left in the bedroom.

How should I bath my baby?

Get organised beforehand. Firstly, *r e l a x*. Your baby can pick up on your anxiety, so keep smiling and give them the very important message that this is fun! You'll need:

- Cotton wool.
- A mild, liquid baby cleanser or bath emollient, such as Weleda (see Resources).
- At least one clean, dry towel. Hooded towels are good for wrapping up your baby from top to toe.
- A clean nappy and clothes.

You only need a shallow bath with enough water to comfortably cover your baby from feet to shoulders.

Never fill a bath with hot water first. It is simply too easy to forget and put your baby in without adding the cold. This can cause serious injury. Check the temperature and check again – it needs to be warm enough that it is comforting but not as hot as you would have as an adult. As a guide, it should be 37–38°C. Buy a bath thermometer if you would like reassurance.

- Bring your baby to the bath area, undress him and remove his nappy. If there's poo in the nappy, clean your baby's genitals and bottom with cotton wool or wipes before putting him in the bath.
- Make sure any doors and windows are closed – babies will feel draughts that we might not.
- Slowly lower him into the water. Remember, he was only recently living in water, so the chances are he will love it. Even small babies will stretch their legs about and wave their hands.

- Support their neck and head on your upturned forearm with your hand holding onto their far arm. With your other hand, support their bottom. They may look startled and unsure; some babies will even try to cling to you. Make them feel safe by keeping a good grip, as they might get quite slippery when wet. Keep smiling!
- Wash your baby's face with clean pieces of cotton wool dipped in warm water and squeezed out.
- If your baby has dried mucus in his eyes or nostrils, dab it first to soften the mucus. Wipe each eye from the nose outwards with a fresh piece of dampened cotton wool.
- Use a mild, liquid baby cleanser to remove any poo, nappy cream and sick that might be trapped in their many lovely folds.
- Use your hand, a flannel or a sponge to clean your baby from top to bottom and from front to back. For your baby's genitals, a routine wash is all that's needed.
- Lift your baby out of the bath, and straight on to a dry towel. Wrap him up warm and pat him dry.
- Just like us, a bath can make a baby thirsty, so offer some breast milk or a bottle afterwards.
- You might want to use this time for a little gentle massage using a suitable oil – olive oil will do, but there are several baby-friendly products on the market without perfumes.
- Put a nappy on and dress your baby ready for their day or for bed. Give them a cuddle to make sure they are still nice and warm.

■ WEEKS FOUR TO SIX: A NEW REALITY

At this time your baby will suddenly seem to 'wake up' – they look around, make more noise and hold their heads up a little stronger. This can be both exhilarating and exhausting. Depending on the nature of your child, he might get bored quite easily and grizzle to be entertained when he is awake. This can be annoying if you feel there are lots of jobs you need to do. So – leave the jobs. Delegate as much as you can and play with your baby. I promise you, this time is much more enjoyable if you can commit to it as a 'job' for a few more weeks at least – don't feel guilty if you spend time 'just' staring at your baby and sticking your tongue out for five minutes until he copies you. It's not always easy, especially if you enjoy intellectual challenges. Look into baby groups and classes where you will get to meet other mums and have conversations with adults. If you had an abdominal birth (**caesarean** – see page 115), this is the time at which you will be insured to drive again, and the chances are you will really enjoy getting this freedom back. Using a sling to carry your baby around can be great at this time. It leaves your arms free for anything you need to do and keeps your baby interested in the world around him. He will love being close to you, hearing your voice and the gentle motion of being carried. But they can make your back ache so a bouncy chair for the kitchen can be a Godsend.

Try playgroups – you will never fail to be amazed at how babies simply love to see other babies. At home, a 'baby gym' is great for buying you a few minutes of peace and giving your baby some mental and physical stimulation. You won't believe how cool it is when they start reaching out for the dangly ladybird and the jingly mirror. This is also the time when meeting up with your antenatal-class friends will be the highlight of your week. Seeing that others are going through the very same stage is the best cure for feeling alone.

If you have healed from the birth and had your six-week check, and your baby has had their immunisations, you can take them swimming. This can be a total joy. Babies love the stimulation of a swimming pool – the noise, the smell and the feeling of being with you in the water are hugely enjoyable for babies. It is also a great way to wear them out so that they sleep well. Make sure to time a swim when they are not hungry or tired. And remember that they will pick up on your feelings – so hide any nervousness you might have with lots of sing-song voices and smiles. Let them see your face and hold them close in the pool.

This is also the time when you can increase your own exercise. Treat yourself to a new pair of trainers and take some longer, medium-paced walks with the pram. This will get your blood pumping, the endorphins flowing and your mood lifted. But if you are breastfeeding, don't attempt any sort of low-calorie diet. Return to the section on **diet** (see page 140) as a reminder to get plenty of vitamins and minerals. Drink plenty of water and even enjoy the odd (well-timed) glass of wine (see **drinking while breastfeeding** page 78).

Postnatal/baby check

Six to eight weeks after the birth, you will be expected to make an appointment at your GP for a postnatal check-up. Your baby will also need checking at eight weeks, so why not make life easy and ask to do both on the same day? Your doctor will check your undercarriage or your abdominal birth scar. They will suggest a smear, but this can give a false positive so soon after birth (and may still sting a little) so decide if you'd rather postpone this. It is entirely up to you.

Your doctor will also want to talk about contraception. Try not to laugh in their face. There are no set rules about getting back in the saddle after birth – if you feel like making love to your partner, then go for it! But remember that you may be fertile while breastfeeding, or even if you haven't had a period. Take things slowly and talk to your partner if you need reassurance. You may need a little extra lube while your hormones settle down, but pain during sex is not inevitable after birth. Visit your GP if you feel any discomfort after 12 weeks.

The very best bit of this first six weeks is that it ends with *smiles* – just when reality has hit. Much of your support network has drifted away and the tiredness has caught up with you, when your baby turns to look at you and *smiles*. And I swear to God, every miserable, tiring and exasperating moment disappears. Suddenly, everything is completely worthwhile.

Y is for . . .

YOU – AND YOUR IDENTITY

Who are you? This is quite an easy question for most women to answer before they've had a baby. We define ourselves by external factors: our profession, our relationship status, hobbies, interests and social life. It's a positive side effect of our modern-day 'me' culture – we've never been so good at knowing what and who makes us happy and aiming for a life that maximises our satisfaction. It's good to be a gal in the twenty-first century.

But postnatal depression is on the rise; survey after survey has dispelled the idea that women can 'have it all', and dilemmas persist every day for women conflicted about returning (or not) to work.

As important as it is to consider birth, breastfeeding and what nappies to use, it's also wise to think a little about how motherhood may change you. The chances are, you'll be surprised that the practicalities will come easily – adjusting to your new (unpaid) job, however, might be harder than you expect.

Don't beat yourself up. Aim low. See **guilt** (page 190). And consider this advice from life coach and mum of Archie, Rebecca Morley:

Rebecca Morley on the new you

In theory, you've had nine months to get your head around becoming a mum, but really nothing can prepare you for the complete and total re-imagination of everything you thought you knew about yourself.

Identity, in coaching terms, is buried deep below the four other levels of our psyche: environment, behaviour, capabilities and beliefs. When you think about the transition to motherhood in these terms, it's no wonder that some new mums struggle. All these four things change with the birth of a baby – many in ways that you couldn't have envisioned.

As not just a coach, but also a recent new mum myself, I've spent a lot of time understanding these changes. Below are my coach–mum thoughts in the hope that they might help you through:

Uncertainty is the new normal
You are, on the whole as an adult, pretty used to knowing the answer to most things. There will be the odd times

when you don't, but, let's face it, they are rarely life or death. Or at least they *were*. Now, on the other hand, you feel as if you don't know anything, and on top of that, what worked yesterday doesn't today. You are not alone. Every mum has felt this way, even the ones who seem to have it completely sorted. Accept that you can't know everything and that no one is expecting you to. Your baby doesn't know any other way. There is no right way to do things and you will get through. The less energy you waste wondering if you're doing a good job, the more energy you'll have to actually do it. And talk, talk, talk to other mums – the best comedy value is definitely not in the success stories – some of my best mum moments so far have been laughing about my worst ones.

Conversation? What conversation?
As soon as you are able to come up for air, you will start to crave adult conversation. Your new social circle will most likely be your antenatal group and, if you're lucky, you'll have more in common than just babies. You might find yourself unable to ever reach the end of a conversation with anyone, as your attention will invariably be swiped by a baby or a monitor. You might go entire days without speaking to anyone but your little bundle of joy. This, as I've found from talking to lots of mums, is one of the most difficult bits to get used to. Why is this? Because talking is our way of processing things, the way we say things makes us who we are. I'd be a fool to try to give you any other advice on this other than to just go with it, get your kicks where you can and make sure your partner knows that you will need to hear about their day, no matter how boring, when they get home.

Your brain will not turn into a ball of mush from misuse, I promise.

Your idea of a mum vs you as an actual mum

You will have, from your upbringing, a pretty fixed idea of what being a mum is all about. The chances are that if your friends and family have had kids, you've made judgements based on these beliefs about whether or not they're doing it right. You will probably also have decided what sort of mum you're going to be, and who you're not going to be like as well. And now you're faced with the reality, and finding out that this is different from what you thought it would be can be a huge blow. Anything that shakes our beliefs is difficult to deal with because they are there for a reason. They give us a framework within which to operate so that every decision in life doesn't take forever. Our beliefs give us psychological breathing space. For someone who is dealing with everything else that comes with being a new mum, this can be one of the most difficult things to deal with. The way you cope with this will have a huge bearing on how you feel ongoing. Seek out and talk to PLMs (people like me). Focus on the people you identify with most now, seek their advice, talk through what you've got going on and ask how they deal with it. And try to embrace the uncertainty if you can, because each time you nail something, your confidence will grow and you'll feel incredible about it.

Identity crisis?

What has become of the person you were before you were expecting? One of my best friends said recently that one of her biggest challenges with becoming a new mum was that no one ever called her by her name any more. She became simply 'Edward's mother'. And along with this comes the fact that suddenly you are judged on the behaviour of another person, one who, despite many people's assertions to the contrary, you have limited control over, especially in the very early days. You also start to realise that all the things you thought you couldn't wait to do again once you'd had the baby suddenly seem a lot less important than they did. All these things relate to the simple, but pretty scary question – who am I? It's not a question we have to ask ourselves very often, and it's not a question that many new mums even know they're struggling with. They just feel a vague but deep-seated sense of uncertainty that they're really not used to. This can affect their relationship with themselves and other people, as they wrestle with this unknown, unfamiliar person they've become.

Be ready to adapt. As you take time to get to know your baby, you also need to take time to get to know the new you. Acknowledge that things have changed, but also think about the things that are still really important to you and make time for them. If it's exercise, for example, get back into it as soon as you possibly can, even if it's just creating a routine that involves a brisk morning walk. The key to balance is about constantly reassessing the different variables and shifting things around to accommodate any changes. Spending a bit of time thinking this through will help you to get there quicker. When it comes to the other stuff, you can try to change the world when you have time again. In the meantime, my advice is just to accept it. There's plenty of time for people to use your name, don't sweat the small stuff!

Z is for ...

ZZZZZ – SLEEP

Alongside poo, sleep is every new parent's favourite topic of conversation. It's a revelation when you realise how many people are walking, driving and working completely sleep deprived at any given moment. Grab naps whenever you can and try to go to bed early – both of which are easier said than done.

Routine

Don't expect your baby to find any sort of routine for the first four to six weeks, no matter what others might suggest. It's totally unrealistic to expect your baby to sleep from 7pm until 7am at this stage (and if you want to breastfeed, it isn't even advisable). You can easily feel like you are 'failing' if you believe this is possible.

For the happiness of most parents, however, it is worth teaching babies the difference between night and day: keep night feeds quiet and dark; daytime should be more lively. Don't feel you have to put your baby in a darkened room for daytime naps – a flexible baby will fit in around your needs (to some extent) and a rigid routine means that you won't be able to go out during their bed-ridden nap times. This may drive you nuts, especially when you see that your antenatal classmates are all meeting for lunch at midday but you need to be at home with your baby in a blacked-out room. In that situation, nobody wins.

Remember that babies cry because they are: hungry, wet, cold, tired, bored or in need of a cuddle. That's it. If there is anything more serious going on healthwise, there are normally other symptoms: a temperature, listlessness or a rash, for example.

If your baby is crying incessantly, take a deep breath and stay calm. If they are dry, fed and cosy, they may simply be crying themselves to sleep. I believe the greatest gift you can give a baby is the ability to self-soothe and put themselves to sleep. This doesn't mean leaving them in a room alone until they stop crying because they have given up on the idea that you will come back. That isn't cool for mum or baby. But I am a great believer in putting your child down to sleep when they are awake, so that they learn to nod off. If they can't self-settle in the day, it's unreasonable to expect them to do so at 3am.

Tired babies rub their eyes, blink slowly and yawn. But it is extremely easy to mistake a crying, sleepy baby for a hungry one. Their innate instincts mean that they may wish to suck themselves to sleep, but as soon as you put them on the breast or offer a bottle they nod off after a few sucks. If you notice your baby doing this, you may want to try some judicious dummy use. But try not to rely on it or you'll spend all night putting it back in!

Dummies are a source of controversy, and rightly so. Few sights make me more bemused than seeing a two-year-old walking around a supermarket with a dummy in its mouth – they aren't developing their speech and have become 'addicted' to the dummy as a crutch. This makes it very difficult for the parent to wean them off. But a well-timed dummy for a sucky baby that you remove once they drop off to sleep is one tool to have in your armoury.

If your baby is refusing to sleep and you feel yourself getting wound up and angry, step back and think: is she hungry? No. Is she wet? No. Is she cold? No. Is she tired? Yes.

So hug them, kiss them and put them down safely in their cot while you go and make a cup of tea. This will be the longest three minutes of your life. But the chances are, they'll be asleep when you come back. If not, give them a quick cuddle, pat them, shush them, offer words of comfort and stroke their head downwards between their eyes for a few seconds. Calm them down. Reassure them and, when they quieten, gently walk out. Return to repeat this reassurance as many times as you need to until they nod off. Eventually, they will recognise the cues of sleeptime and won't need this extra coaching.

Be warned that evenings – between 5.30 and 8pm – can be extremely difficult. Babies wish to cluster-feed, which is a clever evolutionary tool, as they fill their bellies before the long, dark nights set in. They are fractious and difficult to please. You can feel as though you spend hours feeding them and aren't able to put them down for a minute. Babywearing in a sling or having a second pair of hands around at this time can be a godsend – so maybe your partner can return from work early with this in mind.

A gentle bedtime routine that you can try after six weeks

- **5.30–6pm** Half a feed (bottle or boob).
- **6–6.30pm** Bath, massage with oils in dimly lit room, nappy and Babygro for bed.
- **6.30–7.30pm** Second half of feed, winding, gentle talking, preparing your changing basket (see **getting organised** page 292) for the night ahead; reading bedtime stories.
- **7.30pm** Place in bed. Kiss goodnight.

Yes, it really can take two hours to get your baby to bed.

This might seem like a long time, but it can be enjoyable, and you will eventually be able to shorten the feeds or the bath time. You need to take it slowly so that your baby develops a sort of

Pavlov's dog's approach to bed: recognising simple sounds, smells and feelings that tell her sleep is coming soon.

You will work out if this is too late for your baby: some get over-tired and cry hysterically, so they may need to be going down at 7pm, in which case shift everything half an hour earlier.

Persistence is key, and not being tempted to take them back down to sit with you on the sofa when they don't calm down. The happiest mums I know are the ones who develop a gentle but effective bedtime routine in the first three months. It won't always go according to your plan. Teething, illness and growth spurts will throw a spanner in the works from time to time.

What the experts say

I was always a bit sniffy about 'sleep consultants' – the idea that we should pay someone to get our babies to sleep, duh! I'd rather muddle on through and spend the money on wine. But having worked with couples who can feel lost, desperate and with their eyeballs melting due to lack of sleep, I totally get it. Many new families don't have older relatives living nearby to help; they may both work and therefore need to be up and out on a train in the morning; they go online and read 3 million different techniques to try, and weep into their four-shot espresso. They don't need a manual, but they do need confidence. Then, they call Annie Simpson. I love Annie, because she is the first to admit that there is no magic cure to get your baby to sleep through the night (whatever that actually means), and as a mum of three she has been there, done that and possesses the confidence that only comes from emerging out the other side and realising that every stage is just a – er, stage. Annie works with Pam and I on our postnatal course, The Happy Baby Club, and offers her wisdom to parents with babies of all ages.

What does Annie hear most and what does she do?

Annie Simpson on sleep problems

The most common sleep complaints we hear are from tired parents who have read lots of conflicting pieces of advice, who have also tried lots of different things and who don't have much faith that they are ever going to sleep again. This is typically because their baby has never slept well, and while it felt manageable for a while, the tiredness has caught up with them. The other scenario we often see is when a baby has slept well and then, due to illness or jet lag, their sleep habits have changed and they can't seem to get them back on track.

Most parents contact us when their baby is six months old, as they know that at this age they are having solids and should be sleeping through the night. I work with families with toddlers where the sleep issue has become more behavioural so it can take longer to resolve. I also work with families with younger babies who need some gentle guidance around tweaking feed and nap times to make it more manageable and to put some good sleep associations in place.

As a sleep consultant, I look at where families are now and where they would like to be. Then we find a manageable way of getting there. I help families to identify their ideal sleep scenario and how that might change in six months, a year, and so on. If their baby or toddler has become dependent on sleep props to settle, I support the family through the process of changing the sleep habits so that the baby is able to settle independently.

Top sleep tips

Routines can sometimes feel unmanageable for parents,

as they seem too strict. I would recommend finding one that complements your parenting style. We all know that babies sleep best in a dark, quiet room, but sometimes it is more important to meet your tribe and enjoy some time together.

Having a baby is such a huge adjustment, and I would recommend spending the first few weeks getting to know your baby and establishing feeding. As things settle down, I would suggest starting to work towards three-hourly feeds so that, months down the line, your baby isn't still snacking. Some days, it will all work brilliantly, and on others it might all seem to turn to custard.

Before trying to get a baby to sleep through the night, it is important to first look at how well they are feeding and make sure that they are taking the right amount of calories at the right time.

It is equally important to make sure that they aren't waking due to discomfort. Reflux – milk and stomach acid being regurgitated due to an undeveloped digestive system – can cause shrieks of pain and often gets missed, so consider if your baby may be suffering from this and would benefit from treatment.

Finally, it is important that you and your partner discuss how you are going to deal with the nights and make sure you are on the same page. In the middle of the night, when it seems as though the rest of the world is asleep, the doubt can creep in. It is normal to have moments of uncertainty, so be there to support each other through these; consistency is the key to success. Don't lose sight of why you are doing this. Sleep deprivation is a universally recognised form of torture, so the best scenario for any family is that you sleep well.

Resources

Acupuncture Gordana Petrovic can be found at www.acupuncture clinicharleystreet.co.uk/. Look up acupressure points for self-use at www.acupressure.rhizome.net.nz

AIMS The Association for Improvement in Maternity Services makes a big difference to women who need support in making choices relating to their birth. www.aims.org.uk

Baby's position see www.milescircuit.com and www.spinning babies.com

Birth-place choice Where do you want to give birth in your area? See www.which.co.uk/birth-choice

Birth pool liners Hire or buy one online at www.birthpool inabox.co.uk

Breastfeeding support See Le Leche League (www.laleche. org.uk), Best Beginnings (www.bestbeginnings.org.uk) and The Breastfeeding Network (www.breastfeedingnetwork.org.uk). Also try the American sites such as Kelly Mom (kellymom.com) and Jack Newman www.breastfeedinginc.ca/index.php

Breech birth For more information, see Shawn Walker's site, breechbirth.org.uk

Cord clamping For more details, see www.bloodtobaby.com

Diet For more details about Jessica Scott's diet, see www.thenutritionkitchen.co.uk

Doula To find out more, see www.doula.org.uk. For how a doula can help you, see doula.org.uk/research/. For the access fund for vulnerable mothers who cannot afford the doula support they need, see doula.org.uk/doula-access-fund/. Olivia Southey can be found at www.oliviasouthey.com

Down's syndrome These two websites offer a balanced perspective for parents-to-be:
www.arc-uk.org
www.downssideup.com/2015/05/dear-mum-to-be-lets-talk-about-downs.html

Exercise in pregnancy Professor Greg Whyte, author of *Bump It Up*, www.gregwhyte.com

Health visitor and lactation consultant Vanessa is at www.vanessachristie.com

Hormones Get to know your hormone cycle – it can be life-changing. See www.hormonehoroscope.com

Human rights If you feel you need advice or information before your birth from a legal perspective (if, for example, your choices are not being met), contact www.birthrights.org.uk. They are also outstanding if you need legal support post-birth

Independent midwives For a list of independent midwives, detailing what is offered and how to book one, see www.imuk. org.uk

Lactation consultants Don't suffer difficult breastfeeding in silence! Contact a registered, certified lactation consultant. Those offering both NHS and private services can be found at www.lcgb.org, and Chloe can be contacted at www.chloe dymond.com

Miscarriage and stillbirth are traumatic events that need not be endured alone. See The Miscarriage Association (www.miscarriageassociation.org.uk) and Saying Goodbye (www.sayinggoodbye.org) and Sands (www.uk-sands.org) are outstanding

Movement Brilliant advice on monitoring your baby's movements at www.kickscount.org.uk

Obstetrician Professor Donald Gibb now has clinics in the north and south of England. Details can be found at www.thebirth company.co.uk/

Osteopath For more exercises to relieve low-back pain and pelvic girdle pain, see Lisa Opie's website www.osteopath-west.co.uk

Pelvic girdle pain You'll find more about this debilitating condition at www.pelvicpartnership.org.uk

Post-natal depression Your GP or health visitor should be your first port of call, but you can also visit www.pandasfoundation.org.uk to reach out for help

Sickness Extreme nausea in pregnancy is no laughing matter. This website is fantastic: www.pregnancysicknesssupport.org.uk

Skin To help clear spots and pimples in pregnancy, try the all-natural gel containing vitamin B_3, aloe vera and witch hazel, Metazene 5, which is available from the American website Life Link www.lifelinknet.com. You can also use a non-comodogenic tinted moisturiser with SPF, such as La Roche-Posay Anthelios XL Spf 50-plus BB Comfort Cream, which is outstanding. Also try a chemical–manual scrub such as Dermalogica Multivitamin Thermafoliant

Sleep problems See Annie Simpson's website for suggestions to resolve sleep problems, on www.infantsleepconsultants.co.uk

Sleeping babies For the latest evidence-based research into normal sleep patterns for babies and advice on safe-sleep practice see www.isisonline.org.uk

Tongue ties These are increasingly common in new babies and likely to cause feeding problems. The best resource is www.tongue-tie.org.uk

Traumatic birth This is on the rise. If you are finding it hard to recover emotionally or physically, look up www.birthtrauma association.org.uk, and for legal support see www.birthrights.org.uk

Vitamin K Among other topics, this is elucidated at on www. sarawickham.com – a fantastic evidence-based research tool

Weleda This company produces some lovely mild, plant-based, fragrance-free products in its baby range. Particularly useful are Baby Calendula Body Wash, Nappy Change Cream and Baby Oil. You'll find the full range at www.weleda.co.uk